NOURISHING RESILIENCE

NOURISHING RESILIENCE

THE THRIVER'S GUIDEBOOK

Wellbeing practices and inspiration to boost health and resilience in the face of any adversity.

LEAH EVERT

MBA, MS, RD, ACSM-EP

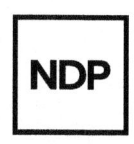

NEW DEGREE PRESS
COPYRIGHT © 2020 LEAH EVERT
All rights reserved.

NOURISHING RESILIENCE

ISBN   978-1-63676-601-0 *Paperback*
        978-1-63676-258-6 *Kindle Ebook*
        978-1-63676-259-3 *Ebook*

This book is dedicated to Thrivers everywhere.

I see you.

I'm proud to be one of you.

CONTENTS

INTRODUCTION 1

PART 1. ADVERSITY AND HOW IT AFFECTS US   **9**

CHAPTER 1. RESILIENCE 11

CHAPTER 2. THE IMPORTANCE OF CONTROL 29

CHAPTER 3. DEALING WITH BLAME 43

CHAPTER 4. POST-TRAUMATIC GROWTH 55

PART 2. PRINCIPLES OF RESILIENCE   **69**

CHAPTER 5. DEFIANCE 71

CHAPTER 6. FINDING PURPOSE 83

CHAPTER 7. COMMUNITY 95

CHAPTER 8. MAKING A DIFFERENCE 107

PART 3. RESILIENCE TOOLS   **115**

CHAPTER 9. NOURISHMENT 117

CHAPTER 10. MOVEMENT 129

CHAPTER 11. MINDSET 135

CHAPTER 12. LOVE 145

CHAPTER 13. KINDNESS 153

CHAPTER 14. AUTHENTICITY 163

CHAPTER 15. BEING BETTER 171

ACKNOWLEDGMENTS 187

APPENDIX 189

INTRODUCTION

"You're not going to die this year, but you probably will next year."

In the spring of 2017, I was one year into business school, six years into my service as a medical officer in the Army Reserves, and ten years into a career I loved. I was also diagnosed with stage four breast cancer and given two years to live.

I was thirty-six years old, and in one moment, my whole life completely changed. I went from planning the life in front of me, which included endless possibilities and the open world ahead, to planning for the end of my life. What did I want to do with my last few years? Should I cash in my 401(k) and travel the world? Or should I continue down the path to a life I'd never lead? In one moment, all my carefully calculated plans and the control I had over my life had completely vanished. I felt powerless and completely incapacitated.

Throughout my life, I'd considered myself an eternal optimist. If something went wrong, I'd search for the bright side or the silver lining. Obviously, this was quite helpful when facing adversity or pain. However, this often didn't allow me to face trials and tribulations in a real way. *Was that a lump on my breast? I don't think so. Could that be cancer? No way, that could never happen to me.*

My internal bright side may have also made me a poor confidant to friends dealing with real pain. After hearing their story, I'd serve up something optimistic, "Cheer up! You'll get past this!" I had no idea that what I was saying wasn't acknowledging real emotions that couldn't, and shouldn't, be tamped down. I was deflecting the suffering instead of looking the pain straight in the face.

When I was first diagnosed with terminal cancer, I didn't absorb what was happening to me. My consistent optimism presented itself as something different: denial. I was too young too healthy too motivated, and too diligent. I'd never be the one sharing big, sad news on Facebook, asking for sympathy, sharing my fears, and counting the days left in my life.

I carried this denial straight through the month-long process to determine the extent of my illness. Biopsies, scans, tests, appointments and appointments and appointments. Each doctor looked increasingly worried as the visits progressed. Nodes involved, extensive liver involvement, what does all this mean?

Finally, one doctor gave it to me straight. "You're not going to die this year, but you probably will next year." It felt like a punch to the gut, which was *exactly* what I needed.

The world is full of adversity. An average of ten million people die of cancer each year. In the US, an estimated forty out of one hundred men and thirty-nine out of one hundred women will develop cancer during their lifetime.[1] Illness, divorce, death, and loss can each cause irreparable damage

---

[1] "Cancer Facts and Figures 2020," American Cancer Society, accessed August 20, 2020.

to our mental health and wellbeing. More than 20 percent of adults are predicted to live with some sort of mental illness, often prompted by a traumatic incident.[2]

When you are faced with adversity, it's easy to become immobilized. When something completely out of your control happens to you—divorce, loss, depression—you're taught to trust others—parents, teachers, doctors, and lawyers. When you're sick, you might shut down and put the control into the hands of your treatment team. However, living with that loss of control can sometimes make you feel worse. Losing your ability to make decisions about your life and health can render you powerless.

But you don't have to be power*less*. You can be power*ful*.

For some, being faced with adversity or a traumatic incident can trigger a perspective that builds strength and self-confidence not found from anything else. Shifting the concept of trauma and adversity to purpose and empowerment can lead to something far more powerful than one has ever experienced, including enlightenment, growth, resolve, and determination.

Four years after that grim prognosis, my perspective has changed completely. I'm actually *thankful* to be living with a terminal illness. I've gained perspective unlike anything I could fathom. Colors are brighter. Experiences are sweeter. Food is tastier. Love is more powerful. Friendships are more restorative. Hope is more contagious.

Even better, worry is fleeting. Stress is trivial. Most problems are inconsequential. My entire outlook has changed for the better.

---

[2] "Learn about Mental Health," Center for Disease Control, accessed August 28, 2020.

This concept, known as post-traumatic growth, is something many people experience after a tragedy or adversity. The individual has experienced something life-altering but also recounts profound changes in their view of relationships, how they view themselves, and their philosophy on life. Individuals who experience this phenomenon all describe growth that was significant *because* of their struggle, not despite it. They equate their subsequent happiness, acceptance, liberation, or validation to their adversity. They're even thankful for it.[3]

For me, I was empowered to *do*. I knew I had to do something productive to make a difference in my life and the lives of others. I'd been a registered dietitian for well over a decade and was a corporate health and wellness consultant for more than forty organizations across the United States, including several Fortune 500 companies. My life's work was to help people feel empowered to be healthy. After my diagnosis, I was startled at how little literature and research there was connecting diet, exercise, and mindset to improved cancer outcomes, complementing their pharmacological treatment plan. However, there were a ton of anecdotes. I received many inspiring stories of hope and struggle. People had beat the odds and had done *something on their own* that may have made a difference. Even though I examined these stories, I couldn't put my finger on the formula for their successes.

I started digging. I had a good understanding of tumor metabolism—how a tumor grows and develops—from years of physiology and biology. I became impassioned about nutrition and exercise and their effect on cellular biology,

---

3 Richard G. Tedeschi and Lawrence G. Calhoun. "Posttraumatic Growth: Conceptual Foundations and Empirical Evidence," *Psychological Inquiry* 15, no. 1 (2004): 1-18.

particularly for metastatic cancer cells. I began to talk to oncologists who included specific lifestyle tools as a part of their practice to determine what could make a difference in the overall outcomes of their patients. They shared with me their pains and told me that studies connecting diet, exercise, and lifestyle to overall survivability rarely got funded because of the inability to patent the outcome.

I decided it was my turn to take control.

In the summer of 2017, my best friend Janine, an exercise physiologist, and I started the Willow Foundation. The Willow Foundation is a nonprofit organization that funds researchers in the areas of diet, exercise, and mindset and measures their impact on late-stage or metastatic cancer patients. Based on our logic, relying on medicine is just not doing enough. Patients need to have some control over their outcome and have the ability to contribute to their care. We believe wholeheartedly that these three things, along with traditional treatment methods, are a key part of the remission equation.

In building the Willow Foundation, I became engrossed even further in the concept of holistic wellbeing. I'd always been a believer in nutrition and exercise as medicine but started to understand the value of other controllable variables. Nutrition, exercise, and mindset were key contributors, but what else could you use to gain some control and feed and grow your resilience?

I began to learn about other cancer patients and survivors of trauma who had an incredible ability to beat dismal odds. Some had been hit with immeasurable adversity and in the end, found their purpose. While most people would crumble, they were stronger *after their adversity*. I found myself drawn to these people who had been faced with the unimaginable and had come out on the other side tougher, more confident, and with more clarity. I talked to these survivors at length about how they'd beaten odds, grown from their adversity, and thrived when others would have wilted. What made these people so resilient? During our conversations, I kept returning to the same concepts, finding commonalities between each of these unique humans. To me, they were more than just survivors, they were Thrivers.

In this book, I share Thriver's stories of hope and survival. I talk to Trevor who had a stroke at the age of thirty and had to relearn how to talk, Nancy who was hit by a car while cycling and given a near-zero chance of recovery, and Stephanie who has a special needs child who is beating all the odds. I'll explore how these special, resilient people have a unique quality: they take charge of their destiny to live full, purposeful lives. While so many of them found their own paths to resilience, one thing remained constant. They were all determined to take their power back.

These conversations and my experience have led me to discover key elements that help us manage adversity, whether illness, injury, or otherwise. I've had countless conversations and have spent years understanding how we can live our best lives and how we can be well. While so much in life is out of our control, I've discovered six things we can do to help us change the trajectory of our lives:

1. **Diet.** Thrivers look at food as nourishment to heal and sustain the body.
2. **Mindset.** Thrivers look at their problems as challenges they *need* to conquer.
3. **Exercise:** Thrivers include movement as a staple component of their life.

4. **Love:** Thrivers find love in unique and special ways.
5. **Kindness:** Thrivers spread goodwill to others.
6. **Authenticity:** Thrivers are liberated by always being their most authentic selves.

Throughout this book, I'll share the ways in which these Thrivers have used the six principles to live full, healthy lives, despite major adversity. We'll dive into the science of these principles to learn what really works and how you can make changes to your everyday life to improve your resilience and grow no matter the size of your adversity. We'll explore how food can be curative, mindset can be restorative, exercise can be soothing, love can be comforting, kindness can be inspiring, and authenticity can be liberating.

This book is for anyone facing adversity in their life—no matter the size. From illness, to divorce, to loss, the stories of these Thrivers and their tenacity and determination to live will motivate you to find purpose. You'll find ways to add determination to your life, just like those in the stories that follow. Their resolve will inspire you, and their habits will help you live a more resilient life. I hope you enjoy my book.

Some names are changed for anonymity.

PART 1

ADVERSITY AND HOW IT AFFECTS US

CHAPTER 1

RESILIENCE

Before cancer changed my life forever, I had a brush with adversity that set me up for a lifetime of resilience. When I was seventeen, I experienced a level of physical pain that was indescribable, which left me searching for answers for more than two years. I was misdiagnosed over ten times. It changed the trajectory of my life. In some ways, it was for the better.

Up until then, I had a typical, loving childhood without trauma, illness, or challenge. My parents did everything in their power to ensure my brother and I grew up normal and happy, and away from adversity. My dad was a career government employee. My mom was home when we were young, but as we got older, she was able to work part time around our schedules. She eventually landed a fifteen-year career with the federal government. Both of my parents were warm, loving people who gave us an equal amount of structure and freedom to grow into ourselves.

Anyone who meets my Dad instantly feels his warmth and joviality. He's the kind of guy who gets along with just about anyone, which I like to think I inherited from him.

He grew up an only child in downtown Baltimore not far from Memorial Stadium, with not much else to do but play outside and listen to Orioles games. He became a lifelong sports fan. Dad played all the sports available to young men back then—football, lacrosse, and baseball. He was a natural.

My mom grew up in the Upper Peninsula of Michigan in a small town on the coast of Lake Superior. Despite the bitterly cold winters, she enjoyed a home filled with warmth with her parents and four siblings. Her mom, my grandmother, centered her entire life around her family. She was the quintessential mother and wife of the time—baking her breads from scratch, maintaining a flourishing garden, and raising five unique, headstrong kids. From a young age, my mom knew she didn't fit into the life of a small-town girl. She wanted more out of life than to live in her slowly progressing, rural town and to simply be a wife and mother, but her aspirations were not encouraged by her parents. At that time, girls in her town were meant to get married, have children, and that's about it.

When my mom was eight years old, she bounded outside to see her brothers playing baseball in the yard. Feeling left out, she demanded to play with them. No one would listen to her. She was only a girl, so her concerns simply didn't matter. She most certainly wasn't allowed to play sports. Determined, my mom walked right up behind her brother as he was mid-swing. *Whack!* The bat hit her just above the right eye. Luckily, her grandmother who lived nearby was a nurse, and she and her grandfather rushed my mom to the hospital.

Despite lots of blood, seven stitches, and one angry mother, my mom was undeterred. While baseball wasn't in the cards, she begged her parents for a season ski pass to the local hill and even worked there after school to pay for her own equipment. She's has been conquering mountains ever since. Later, she taught herself how to play tennis too. Even at seventy years old, she still plays twice a week. She and my dad made sports and fitness a huge part of their lives, and credit it to their good health and strong marriage. It only made sense that my life would become centered around sports too.

When asked what I wanted to be when I grew up, I always answered, "Professional athlete." My young life was built around tennis matches, softball games, soccer practice, and dive team meets. My entire identity was hitched to my ability to thrive in sports. By the time I was in high school, I was being recruited to play both tennis and softball in college. In fact, it was pretty much my only determining factor when searching for colleges. During my senior year of high school, I was on my way to my ultimate goal, as a handful of colleges were vying for my attention. Everything was looking up until I was hit with the worst pain I could ever imagine.

The sun beamed down on the tennis court, creating a gorgeous fall day in Virginia. I had just begun my senior year of high school and was playing on my school's tennis team. I loved the sport. The competition thrilled me, and the team camaraderie pushed me to be better. The matches were always exhilarating. I relished in the feeling of my racket smacking the ball, having the precision to place it where I wanted on my opponent's side of the court. Each point, each game won contributed to our team's overall chances of winning our district, bringing us one step closer to the state tournament.

On this beautiful fall day, I strutted out to the court on my home turf. We had fans surrounding the courts, including my friends and family. I began the match confidently and was soon knee-deep in a tough battle against a local adversary.

We were neck-and-neck when I went on offense. I went up for a serve. Suddenly, a sharp, searing pain stabbed me in my neck. The pain cascaded up into my head and down my arm, and I collapsed into a heap on the court. My family rushed to collect me, but after a few minutes, the pain had subsided. I was okay. *What was that?*

Over the next few months, the pain returned: always sporadically, but not always during movement. The pain was so intense it would wake me up at night or keep me from playing sports. I could never predict its onset because it was so random. I started to try anything and everything to mitigate the pain—daily ibuprofen, prescription opioids, neurologists, physical therapists, massage therapists, orthopedists. Everyone was stumped. The pain was too sporadic to be diagnosed properly. Each person had a different theory. One doctor thought I had muscle spasms. Another thought it was bone degeneration. No one thought it was of any major concern.

However, time progressed and I failed to recover. I finished high school and the pain had gotten progressively worse. I started college and the pain became more frequent. In almost two years, I had over fifty incidents like the first one, with isolated bouts of searing, debilitating pain. I was failing classes because I couldn't sleep through the night. I was beginning to think I'd never have relief.

In the spring of my freshman year, my mom made me an appointment with a renowned neurosurgeon named Dr. Hope. This was it. For some reason, I finally felt some optimism, and I couldn't discount the excitement I felt after simply learning his name. Dr. Hope was supposed to be a master diagnostician and could help people who hadn't been able to find relief from past therapies. Finally, I thought, it was my turn.

Dr. Hope had me bring my X-rays and most recent magnetic resonance images (MRIs) to his office to do an exam. He spent a few minutes with me, checking my mobility and massaging my pain-inflicted area. He tried to recreate the pain I'd describe, but it was so random and sporadic that it wasn't possible. After a few minutes, he looked me square in the eye. "Nothing is wrong with you, my dear," he stated, his tone dripping with condescension. "I won't do any surgery when you're completely healthy."

My nineteen-year-old, exhausted face tilted up at him and tears spilled down my face. Never in my life did I so desperately want something to be wrong with me. Deep down, I knew this pain wasn't fabricated. Something was causing this catastrophic effect on my body. He looked at my tears, smiled, and said, "Crying is not going to help you." He made it clear that he thought I was simply a malingering patient, grossly overexaggerating my pain. With that, he left the room. Dr. *Hope* had left me with none.

I've thought about that moment many times over the years. I've pondered over how one person's judgment of my health and my body could have been the end of me. I was on the edge, struggling in school, in enough pain that I couldn't see the road ahead. I was stuck, frozen in time, paralyzed with the what-next. Here it was, the end of my road. *Nothing wrong with me. Keep downing the pills. Stop complaining.* It had been almost two years of accepting my fate, and Dr. Hope had finally sealed it. This was my life now.

Luckily, my mom didn't see it that way. With the same determination she brought to the ball field as an eight-year-old, she made it her personal mission to find a diagnosis that fit my symptoms. The internet was still relatively new at that time, but she went to Google to find something that matched.

Deep within her search, she came upon a neurosurgeon who worked on patients with a rare brain malformation that seemed to cause symptoms similar to mine.

Could this obscure structure issue be the key to my pain? She called his office and begged for me to be seen. This physician was extraordinarily busy and only took referrals from other doctors. But my mom was persistent, pouring her heart out to the receptionist while trying to make an appointment. Luckily, she took pity on my mom and scheduled me in. Hope was beginning to be restored. Dr. Weingart was a hot commodity and world renowned for this kind of brain malformation.

A few weeks later, we met Dr. Weingart. He took one look at my MRI and confirmed it. Yes, I had Chiari Malformation—a condition where the brain tissue extends into the spinal canal. It occurs when part of the skull is abnormally small or misshapen, pressing on the brain and forcing it downward. It can cause pain and can be dangerous if it blocks the flow of cerebral spinal fluid.

Despite the diagnosis, I'd never been so relieved. My mom, my hero for her persistence and forever faith that my pain was true, broke down in tears. I couldn't believe how happy we were to find out my brain was malformed. Sure, my brain was a mess, but I was simply delighted! Dr. Weingart, however, wasn't totally convinced the malformation was causing my pain. Since my pain was only on one side of my head, he hypothesized that I might have a rare condition, something he'd only seen once before in his twenty-five-year career. He asked me to do one more test, a bone scan, to rule it out.

One week later, my bone scan came back, and Dr. Weingart was right. In addition to my brain malformation, I had a large, growing bone tumor on my cervical spine, pressing against my spinal column. Dr. Weingart explained it was the likely cause of my pain, not the malformation, and we'd need to do surgery to remove it as soon as possible. I couldn't believe it. How could all of those doctors, including Dr. Hope, have missed both of these diagnoses? Luckily, we finally had a game plan and moved quickly. Within a week, I had surgery to remove the tumor.

The surgery was invasive, and I was in the hospital for several days. I woke up with a brace strapped tightly around my neck and was instructed to keep it on for three straight months. The doctors had removed the tumor with clear margins, and all I had to do now was heal. I was completely relieved. After I returned home from the hospital, I endured a long, boring summer filled with books and movies and not a lot of movement. But by the end of the summer, I healed up enough to get back to playing sports. Most importantly, I was pain-free.

My experience of unrelenting pain helped me understand the importance of resilience in a person's life. Resilience is a common phrase these days, something we all talk about needing to manage the pains of daily life. Back when I was suffering, however, resilience wasn't such a catchy word. If you were in pain, you were admired for toughing it out. Admitting something was wrong wasn't really an option. However, there's no bouncing back if you don't acknowledge the root of the pain in the first place.

I've grown to learn a lot about resilience, and how important it is to acknowledge pain and build the mental muscles to manage it, despite adversity. Because I grew up without a lot of adversity, my resilience muscles didn't really grow until I was hit with real pain. Resilience, by definition, is the ability to mentally or emotionally cope with a crisis or to return to pre-crisis status quickly.[4] This doesn't mean ignoring your hardship. This means actually dealing with issues and adversity and developing a plan to manage their outputs. Resilient people develop strength for all kinds of stressful situations and are able to mitigate the rise of overwhelming emotions. However, there are a lot of ways to develop resilience that don't include getting a tumor on your spine. Resilience is a muscle that can be strengthened over time by increasing vulnerability, recognizing emotions, pausing in the heat of the moment, and thoughtfully reflecting on emotional experiences.[5] Each person has the power to grow their resilience through stressful times, despite the level of adversity they may face.

One of the most inspiring stories of resilience is that of my friend, Trevor. In 2012, Trevor was living the young professional's dream. He was twenty-eight years old and had just gotten married. He and his new bride lived in downtown Manhattan, and he had a job working for a large investment bank on Wall Street. Trevor's life was right on track: an Ivy League education, a new family in the works, and a great job.

"Nothing was in the way of a great life ahead," he said. "I felt like everything was going exactly as planned."

Late in the year, Trevor started to endure some pain in his stomach. Shortly thereafter, he noticed increasing blood in his stool. He knew something wasn't right, but he couldn't understand why this was happening to him. He ate a normal diet and never had gastrointestinal issues before. Soon, he started to have regular flare-ups.

Not only were they painful, but these incidents started to change his daily life. One minute, he'd be in a meeting,

---

4 "Building Your Resilience," *American Psychological Association* (blog), 2012, accessed May 15, 2020.
5 Ibid.

the next he'd be running into the bathroom. Some days, he'd go to the bathroom more than twenty times. Finally, he went to the doctor and was diagnosed with ulcerative colitis. He started regular treatment immediately. Things started to normalize.

Trevor learned ulcerative colitis is an autoimmune disorder that causes your body to attack healthy tissue. In Trevor's case, his colon was constantly inflamed, and he was managing regular pain. The drugs were starting to help, but the flare-ups continued. Trevor, however, was tough. A former division one football player, he knew how to push through adversity. He could manage this.

Over time, however, the flare-ups worsened. In fact, a few times, Trevor even required hospitalizations for his colitis. He went through multiple bouts of IV steroid treatments. The treatments were helpful but didn't come without issues. Every time he went through a steroid treatment, his immune system weakened, leaving him at risk for other illnesses. It also magnified mood swings, and the emotional stress he endured started to put a strain on his marriage. But Trevor persisted. He kept working despite regular, painful episodes. He was determined to live his life the way he'd planned. In fact, in early 2014, he and his wife got pregnant and had their first child, a happy, healthy boy.

A few months later, Trevor and his wife went away for the weekend to visit family in upstate New York for the long Easter weekend. The visit was lovely, and Trevor hated to leave. His wife and young son were going to stay upstate a bit longer. However, toward the end of the trip, Trevor started to endure some increasingly annoying headaches. Despite this, he insisted he needed to return to the city to get back to work on Monday morning. He took the train back to Manhattan and returned to his apartment. When he went to bed, he noticed the headache just wouldn't quit. In fact, it was starting to get worse. Trevor shrugged it off, assuming he simply needed a good night's sleep.

The next morning, Trevor awoke with a shock. He looked around. The entire room was spinning. For a few moments, he wasn't quite sure where he was. Eventually, he regained his composure and realized he was all alone in his apartment in New York. The headache from the night before had gotten substantially worse. Something was definitely wrong. He was by all means a normal, active thirty-year-old man. Despite his intestinal flare-ups, he was in good health. Could that have anything to do with his head?

Trevor wrestled with the idea of skipping work. He could roll over, stay in bed, ditch the office, and sleep it off. Perhaps some Advil would put the pain at bay. Somehow Trevor knew this was more serious than just a headache. After a few minutes of uncertainty, he put himself in a cab and went directly to the emergency room.

That one decision saved his life. The increasing pain in his head was substantially more than just a headache. Soon after arriving at the hospital, Trevor had a major stroke. When he went for an MRI, doctors found three large clots in the left frontal lobe of his brain requiring immediate treatment. These clots had originally formed in his colon due to his colitis. The clots had broken off and clogged the blood flow to his brain. This catastrophic event was extremely rare, especially for a young, otherwise healthy colitis patient.[6]

---

6   Deepak Joshi et al., "Stroke in Inflammatory Bowel Disease: A Report of Two Cases and Review of the Literature," *Thrombosis Journal* 6, no. 2 (March 21, 2008).

If Trevor hadn't been at the hospital, he almost certainly would have died. If he had decided to stay home and try to go back to sleep, he would have had a major stroke alone in his apartment and no one would have been around to assist him or call for help. To this day, Trevor isn't sure why he thought this particular headache warranted a trip to the ER, but that one decision undoubtedly saved his life.

Trevor doesn't remember much about the following week. He knows he was in the hospital's intensive care unit. He knows he endured a significant amount of swelling to his brain and the doctors had trouble getting the swelling down. Trevor recalls, "Your brain is like a balloon with a bike helmet on top. There's only so much expansion it can tolerate."

Right after Trevor's stroke, his brain swelled exponentially. In fact, the swelling was so out of control that Trevor's care team was less than an hour away from performing a last-resort brain surgery that would have potentially saved his life but would have undoubtedly left him with major brain damage. Luckily, the drugs finally started working and Trevor's brain swell reduced significantly. He was able to avoid further brain damage.

Unfortunately, Trevor didn't escape unscathed. Despite avoiding additional brain damage, the three clots and subsequent blood loss to his brain had wreaked havoc on his body. Upon waking, Trevor realized he didn't have function or control of the entire right side of his body, from head to toe. He also couldn't speak. No one on his care team could tell him whether any of those functions would ever return. In fact, they estimated Trevor would endure years of treatment and therapy and would never regain his previous strength. In one instant, Trevor's life had forever been changed.

When Trevor awoke from his stroke, he realized very quickly that he was virtually motionless. Even more disconcerting, he couldn't speak. "It turned out I had aphasia," he told me. "I wasn't able to form thoughts and sentences in my brain, but when tasked with making a sound, my brain couldn't signal to my lips and throat to verbalize words." He was completely frustrated and demoralized. Immediately, the therapists in his rehab hospital started to work on him in a way they thought he'd respond—by treating him like an athlete. Each day, they'd set goals for him, starting with simple movements and sounds.

For the next few months, Trevor worked with his coaches—physical therapists, occupational therapists, and speech therapists—to see if he could make any improvement in his movement and his speech.

"It was like going back to first grade English class," he recounted. "I had to learn how to say words and spell words and even how to put a sentence together again." Here he was, an Ivy League star, a Wall Street go-getter, and he was going back to elementary school. "It was beyond maddening for me," he said. "At times, I just wanted to put my head through the wall."

Trevor's prognosis was never clear. His doctors were not optimistic that he'd regain function in his right side or that his speech would return to normal. From the first time he woke, however, Trevor knew in his heart that he'd most certainly walk and talk again. The stroke and subsequent illness themselves had become tangible obstacles to conquer. His determination to return to normalcy was immediately intact. Walking and talking was something he simply *had* to do.

Trevor's bout with adversity was undoubtedly difficult to manage. He was, by all accounts, a healthy, normal human.

But his brush with death did, inadvertently, change his perspective on life and has improved his ability to manage and deal with smaller bouts of adversity. Adversity is often perceived as negative and as something someone has to endure. But adversity and struggle have the power to unify and empower people and truly build resilience. In times of trouble, family members, communities, and even nations band together to provide support to overcome struggles together. Adversity can bring out the best in the world.

In addition, adversity is one of the most powerful mechanisms for personal growth. As some people try to *remove* adversity from their worlds, their ability to *manage* future bouts diminishes. In reality, when you take away adversity, you take away one of the most powerful ingredients to human growth. In fact, a fair number of researchers have delved into the science of adversity and resilience over the past twenty years. Initially, research into resilience mostly focused on the psychological and physical characteristics that were thought to be protective in the face of adversity. In 2002, Dr. Glenn Richardson at the University of Utah started to look at resilience as determined not only by personal characteristics but also by the wider experiences of that person. He determined resilience could be learned if practiced.[7]

Practicing for resilience without adversity requires time and attention. All people, despite their level of trauma, could benefit from behavioral therapy to work on emotions and stress management techniques because we all deal with adverse events daily. By learning how to diffuse tough situations quickly, reducing catastrophic thinking, dealing with counterproductive beliefs, cognitive problem-solving, and

---

7   Romeo Vitelli, "Learning to be Resilient," *Psychology Today*, May 13, 2013.

developing strong social support, we can bolster resilience exponentially and better prepare ourselves for any major trauma of the future.[8]

In addition, Dr. Jane Gilgun at the University of Minnesota at Twin Cities found that the most resilient people had experienced multiple risks over their lives by giving them a set of skills to deal with current adversities. These people were able to draw on social and individual resources to manage adversity, relying on specific, controllable tools that could, in turn, mitigate the stress in their daily life. The interesting part is that the learned resilience doesn't matriculate due to large, catastrophic events. Your resilience can be built on small, daily struggles that each of us endures. What builds your resilience is your ability to acknowledge your emotions authentically and slowly build a mindset that views obstacles as challenges, puzzles needing completing, or mountains needing summiting.[9]

Before my tumor experience, I had no idea how to manage adversity. Until that point in my life, my most significant struggle was my ongoing feud with my brother or some bullying from the girls in school. However, I often catastrophized these events, despite how innocuous they were. I wasn't resilient. Every small adverse event caused ripples in my life from which I could not recover. I was quick to react and quick to feel. I'd always been a sensitive kid, someone who felt more than others. Things stuck with me for a very long time, and I mulled over adversity and conflict for days. Suddenly, I was faced with something that was truly terrifying and life altering. It seemed as though my mindset had shifted.

---

8   Richard G. Tedeschi and Lawrence G. Calhoun, ibid.
9   Steven M. Southwick et al., "Resilience Definitions, Theory, and Challenges: Interdisciplinary Perspectives," *European Journal of Psychotraumatology* 5, no. 1 (October 2014): 25338

I look back at those two years of excruciating bouts of suffering and I believe my ability to withstand my pain and endure consistent doubt and uncertainty helped to define my character. I was still young but started to feel a sense of maturity I hadn't experienced before. Immediately, I started to feel grateful for my experience. This was a true test of my resilience. Minor irritants began to pale in comparison to my tumor diagnosis and subsequent months of immobility, and I was able to have a more tempered view of adversarial situations.

During this time, I made two promises to myself. First, I was never going to let anyone convince me that what I was feeling wasn't true. My experience with Dr. Hope had been demoralizing. Although I understood him to be a brilliant surgeon, his steadfastness on my assured normal health was morally wrong and incompetent. I knew in my heart something was wrong with me. I just needed to find someone who believed in me. Luckily, for me, that was my mom.

Second, I decided to own my health. I majored in Exercise Science. I received a master's degree in Sports Nutrition and Exercise Science and became a Registered Dietitian and Exercise Physiologist. I knew traditional medicine, while powerful, was not the be-all-end-all of human health. I became passionate about the healing movement and food as fuel. I also became empowered by learning about polyphenols and antioxidants that can help stunt chronic illness, reverse disease, and heal bodies. I was hooked on the empowerment this field was able to give me.

Little did I know that this first brush with adversity was nothing compared to the tsunami I would deal with seventeen years later. This experience gave me the boost I needed to start building my resilience skills and the motivation I needed to take a hold of my life.

Trevor also endured a catastrophic event that changed his life for the better. His story really resonated with me because I knew his stroke quite obviously affected him deeply, but it also changed his outlook on life in several ways. I'd known him to be a quiet, introspective person who loved sports, God, and his family. However, Trevor was also a hard charger, driven to accomplish things in life. He'd been on the perfect track. He had a great job, a new marriage, and a young son. His life as he knew it, and expected it, had been completely disrupted in an instant.

After his stroke, Trevor told me that he never returned to his previous "normal." In retrospect, Trevor realized he was living a life in need of some serious adjustments. "I was always internalizing my stress," he said, "Instead of dealing with or managing my issues, I'd simply not talk about it."

Trevor was the kind of person who kept things to himself, didn't talk about problems, and didn't admit to having stressors. After his stroke, Trevor gained a clarity he admitted he'd otherwise never have. The pain and struggle he endured to come back from near death allowed him to become a more authentic person, be open with his feelings, and connect with others on a deeper level. Because of his stroke, he feels more empathy toward others, enjoys a deeper connection with his friends, and has placed a higher emphasis on his relationship with his family.

Trevor did, however, thrive through his rehab. With daily work, he was able to slowly get back to walking. Soon, he was able to form words. Eventually, they turned into sentences. Sometimes he'd struggle to find the right words and his overwhelming journey seemed insurmountable. But he kept after it. After three months, he finally left the hospital, able to walk again. A few months later, he was able to run. Within a year, he was back to working on Wall Street. He even had a new baby girl on the way.

Trevor's story is astounding to me.

"If I had to put a number on it, I'd say I'm back to about 95 percent."

The stroke caused deficiencies in his health that will never be repaired. But he thinks he's pretty close. His humbling experience of deficiency has caused him to see life in a completely different light. When rehabbing, he saw many people who had been hit with a similar fate and weren't able to regain the use of their extremities. Some even died. He realized how fragile life is and how important it is to prioritize the things most important to him: his family and his faith. His adversity had awakened him to a whole new perspective. Despite all his adversity, he believes his stroke made him a better man. He believes he is stronger because of it. *This* is resilience.

CHAPTER 2

THE IMPORTANCE OF CONTROL

I never thought my search for the perfect bra would be the catalyst for an entirely different life.

I had just returned from a ski trip in Colorado and was packing a little bit too much into my busy schedule. Suddenly, I realized my friend's birthday party was only one day away, and I needed a great outfit. I had a dress I thought would work but didn't have the right bra to go with it. This party was a pretty big event, and I'd definitely know most of the attendees. I only had one day to find something that would work.

Desperate, I searched online for a lingerie store that was walking distance from my condo in the Adams Morgan neighborhood of Washington, DC. I relished the excitement in the air of the impending improving weather on this gorgeous spring day. March always felt like anticipation in DC. People were slowly emerging from their winter cocoons, even more prominent on the busy, buzzy streets of my neighborhood.

Soon enough, I found my store. I scaled the flight of stairs to the top of the townhouse converted into small, locally owned stores and entered with some trepidation. I was immediately in awe. I couldn't simply peruse the items because it was one of those high-end lingerie stores. Here, you had to be fitted professionally, and the bras would run you somewhere between $60 and $250 each. Exorbitant, but decadent. For the past twenty-five years of my life, I'd always bought bras without assistance. I knew my girls—what I liked, what was comfortable, what made me feel good. In fact, the thought of someone telling me how to look sexy somehow felt disingenuous. But I was desperate; the party was fast approaching.

I started to look around, my judgment waning. Stephanie, the owner, approached me cautiously. *What did I like? What was I into? How did I want to feel?* I immediately liked her style. I connected with the female empowerment that seemed to ooze not only from Stephanie but also from the store's decor and displays. Sure, you could buy crotchless panties, but they were made from French lace, so they *must* be classy. I loved that Stephanie seemed to immediately *get* me. She helped pick out items that she knew would match my persona and make me look fabulous. Suddenly, my need for a new bra turned into a desire for many new pieces of stunning lingerie.

In the middle of my fitting, Stephanie stopped and looked at me in the mirror. "Your left breast is larger than your right, did you know that?" I did. I told her it'd been that way my entire life. "Really? The way I am measuring, it's almost a cup size different." I looked in the mirror, one with the words "self-care" written in beautiful script across, and took a closer look. She was right. How long had it been like this, and how hadn't I noticed?

As I walked home, I thought about my medical routines. I had just been to the gynecologist in December, which was only three months ago. She'd done a breast exam then, right?

I remember her saying everything looked great. I was only thirty-six, four years away from routine mammograms. *Is there something I missed?*

Once I returned home, I examined myself more closely. Stephanie was right. I pressed more deeply on the top of my skin and noticed the distinctness. A lump was growing in my left breast, making for a noticeable difference in fullness. I felt it more carefully with my right hand. I couldn't have been more confident: it was most certainly a fast-growing, fluid-filled cyst.

A week went by and my breast lump continued to grow. I remember reading about breast cancer, and how the riskiest lumps grow slowly and are often attached to the breast wall. This lump was big and fleshy and close to my skin. Regardless, it seemed to grow by the day, so I made an appointment to see my primary provider. She took a quick look and asked me to get an ultrasound. "It's probably nothing," she said, "but you'll want to do it for peace of mind."

Less than a week later, I proceeded to the radiologist's office for my appointment. Overly confident about the state of my lump, I went to the appointment alone. The radiology assistant began the ultrasound, and our small talk and chatter slowed as she slid the wand across the top of my left breast. I peeked over to the screen and saw what looked like dense, dark striations among the tissue. "I'm going to get the radiologist to take a look, okay?" My heart lurched. Something was wrong.

My radiologist was a tough, no-nonsense kind of woman. She came into the room and took charge of the machine. Quickly, she retraced the scanned area the tech had just completed and looked down at me, "Well, I can tell you this. It's not a cyst. And to be honest, I'm really worried."

That moment is seared into my brain. *How did I let this happen? Had I not been paying attention? Was I not being healthy enough? What could have brought this on? Could it be that I have cancer?* I had virtually no family history of cancer, let alone breast cancer, which is one of the most hereditary types. Both my grandmothers had lived well into their nineties. I was a Registered Dietitian, and I was committed to a healthy lifestyle. I ate "cleaner" than most people I knew. I was too young, too active, too healthy. *How could this be happening?* I left her office feeling numb. I got into my car and immediately called my best friend, Janine. "Don't worry. We'll figure it out, no matter what," she said. I then called my parents, who told me to come over immediately. We sat at the table for hours contemplating our next steps.

"I know women who don't have children are more likely to have breast cancer," my mom reminded me. I'm sure she was not trying to make me feel worse, but it stung. I had heard this statistic before. Women who have their first child at age thirty-five or younger tend to get an overall protective benefit against breast cancer.[10] Despite this, I never thought it would happen to me. My logic or, rather, my naiveté, had me believe that women with breast cancer were generally older than me, were more likely to be overweight, had a family history, or didn't take care of themselves in some way. I had been unlucky in love so far and unable to find a partner with whom to start a family, so my penance was to be diagnosed with cancer? *How could the world be doubly cruel?*

Over the next few weeks, I was ferried in a haze to appointments, discussing my options with surgeons,

---

10 "Does Pregnancy Affect Breast Cancer Risk and Survival?" *Komen Perspectives* (blog), January 2012, accessed September 6, 2020.

oncologists, fertility specialists, and more. I went through countless tests—a bone scan, computed tomography (CT) scan, MRIs, multiple biopsies, and so on. Just when I was getting the strength to manage my new normal—considering the option of losing my breasts and dealing with the onslaught of breast cancer treatments—I hit a new low. I received the call from my oncologist while I was in the car with Janine on our way to the hospital.

"Leah," she said, "the spots we saw on your liver on the CT scan have come back as cancer, the same type that was in your breast. I'm sorry, this means the cancer has spread. At this point, there's no reason to do surgery. We're just going to have to do our best with medicine to keep this contained as long as possible."

I've never felt the weight of something hit me as hard as in that moment. Until then, I had felt ready and prepared. Breast cancer was one of the most curable cancers. I had heard so many stories of "survivors" who were able to have surgery, manage a course of radiation, and maybe lose their hair while undergoing chemotherapy. Some were back in action within a year. What about "save the ta-tas," and all the other trite, overly positive campaigns lightening the reality of breast cancer? Yes, it was prolific. Yes, one in eight women would get it in their lifetime, but most of them would eventually get better.[11] Was she really telling me I was terminal?

At my next appointment, I clarified my new reality. "Am I going to die from this?" I asked her.

"Yes," she said plainly.

"What's the average lifespan?" I asked.

---

11   "Risk of Developing Breast Cancer," BreastCancer.org, accessed September 6, 2020.

"About two years," she replied.

"Is there anything I can do to change that?" I was spiraling, and I needed some control.

"We don't know enough about how lifestyle affects outcomes, but it makes sense to eat healthy and to keep exercising." The feeling of control or having a say over what happens to you in your life is incredibly important for a person's mental health and wellbeing. Researchers have found that having a sense of control increases overall happiness but can even have an effect on mortality rate. Judith Rodin, a former psychologist at Yale University, explains that empowering end-of-life patients with the ability to make even trivial decisions about their care can greatly improve psychological wellbeing as well as potentially extend their life expectancy.[12]

Perceived control is an individual's perception of his or her ability to bring about desired outcomes and prevent undesirable ones. Many patients dealing with cancer have to balance perceived control with items outside of their control. Lifestyle variables, such as nutrition, exercise, kindness toward others, and vulnerability are tools that have a proven value in a person's health and wellbeing. However, it's important to weigh these variables with the reality that there are many things, such as side effects, drug effectiveness, and other people's opinions, which are out of their control. Striking this balance is challenging, but it can be an effective way to empower those facing adversity.[13]

---

[12] E. J. Langer and J. Rodin, "The Effects of Choice and Enhanced Personal Responsibility for the Aged: A Field Experiment in an Institutional Setting," *Journal of Personality and Social Psychology* 43, 2 (1976).

[13] Francisco Pagnini, Katherine Bercovitz, and Ellen Langer, "Perceived Control and Mindfulness: Implications for Clinical Practice," *Journal of Psychotherapy Integration* 26, 2 (2016): 91-102.

A broad range of studies conducted over the past fifty years suggests that perceived control is an important construct for physical health and psychological wellbeing. When people feel they can exert control, they demonstrate better immune responses, cardiovascular functioning, physical strength, increased longevity, increased life satisfaction, and decreased anxiety and depressive symptoms. Feeling like you have a say in your outcomes has a profound effect on your resilience.[14]

Nancy, the mother of my friend Adam, knows all too well how important it is to have control in her life. In 2019, Nancy and her husband spent a month in Florida enjoying the balmy February mornings in the sunshine state. Nancy, a multiyear world champion triathlete was preparing for the Fort Lauderdale Las Olas triathlon. Each year, she spent countless hours of training. The prior year, as a seventy-year-old, she won her age group in the United States Olympic distance triathlon championships. Later, after joining Team USA, she raced at the world championship in Australia and snagged the bronze medal. Nancy was at the very top of the sport. These three sports were some of the most important things in her life.

In typical fashion, Nancy was hustling through a training ride on her bike. "I was out front, my husband was behind me because, well, I'm faster," she said, and laughed. She was clipped into her race bike, effortlessly navigating the traffic on the moderately busy street. Not far into the ride, they entered a roundabout. Seemingly out of nowhere, a car came racing through the yield sign at breakneck speed. Nancy doesn't remember what happened next, but her husband watched with sheer horror. The reckless driver didn't see

---

14 Ibid.

Nancy and struck her with such force that she and the bike, clipped together via her shoes, sailed through the air. She landed headfirst on the pavement, sixty feet from the impact, and her bike helmet cracked in two.

Nancy's husband rushed to her side. She was laying there, unconscious in a pool of blood. Immediately, he questioned whether she was alive. A group of bystanders started to gather, offering immediately to act as witnesses. They had seen what happened and would testify if they needed to. The driver was distracted, didn't see Nancy, and was completely at fault.

Nancy was airlifted to the closest hospital. Luckily, the hospital crew was able to stabilize her. She was alive, but she remained unconscious.

Nancy's family raced to her side, and they were met with a series of unknowns. Nancy was unconscious, undergoing assessments and tests to determine her fate. Nancy's sister-in-law, a nurse, wasn't optimistic. Coma patients are measured extensively to understand the likelihood of recovery. The measurement includes eye opening, verbal responses, and motor responses. The score is provided in the range of 3 to 15. When a patient is scored at 15, it indicates that he or she has a very good chance of fully recovering. A score of 3 provides the patient with the worst prognosis. Scores between 3 and 5 are potentially fatal. Nancy scored a 4.[15]

The intensive care unit (ICU) team, as well as Nancy's sister-in-law, assumed almost no chance that Nancy would recover from her injury. Even if she did live through the coma, her chance of waking up at all was next to never.

---

15 "What Is the Glasgow Coma Scale?" *BrainLine* (blog), February 13, 2018, accessed August 30, 2020.

A week later, against all odds, Nancy miraculously woke from her coma. The critical care staff was utterly shocked. "No one thought I'd wake up. The ICU staff were the most surprised people in the room," Nancy shared. Everyone was dumbfounded at how she had beaten the odds, but Nancy wasn't. "I knew it was because of my fitness level that I was able to survive." Even though Nancy awoke, she had a tough road ahead of her. Not only could she not walk, but there were parts of her body she couldn't even move.

After her stint in critical care, Nancy moved to a rehabilitation hospital with hopes of regaining strength and mobility. There, Nancy started an intense rehab routine. *This is going to be a long, hard journey,* she thought, frustrated that she'd gone from being in the best shape of her life to not being able to move her toes. Something about the challenge piqued her determination. "Right there, at that moment, I knew I was going to work hard and make it back."

By April, Nancy started to see some progress. She could move her legs and stand, but she still couldn't walk. Her family was by her side the entire time, including her son, Adam, and his fiancée, Rachel. A year prior, Adam had given Nancy hip-hop dance lessons for Christmas, which they attended together. Both liked to dance and were excited about their mother-son dance at his wedding. So Nancy started to visualize that day. As soon as she could talk, she said to Adam, "I'm going to dance at your wedding in September, I promise."

Nancy had set her goals. She knew exactly how to work hard and what it feels like to train every day. "So, that's simply what I decided I was going to do."

Nancy returned home determined to thrive despite her new challenges. She set up her rehab schedule, got the right medical support, and was eventually able to move, eat, and walk, albeit with a cane, on her own. Eventually, her therapists said she had graduated. Never did they think Nancy would survive such a tragedy, let alone thrive enough to walk. They were thrilled, and based on their measurements, their work was done. They told Nancy they'd gotten her as far as she could go. Nancy was bewildered. Sure, she could walk, but she couldn't do much else. She couldn't run, she couldn't move her left shoulder. Did they really think she'd be satisfied with that? Nancy became immediately determined. The time had come to take control of her own health.

When someone has faced an accident or traumatic incident, it's easy to feel like their life has been taken from them. They may feel shock, anger, guilt, or even have trouble believing it happened. In addition, many who have dealt with a traumatic incident keep going over the event in their mind. Reliving it helps them try to make sense of it, if possible.

Despite this, there's a lot they can't control when it comes to managing illness, side effects of an accident, or trauma. It can feel difficult to relinquish responsibility for the things they can't control. However, research suggests that if they're able to transfer their loss of control over the incident to items which they can, they'll be better at improving mental wellbeing, coping with trauma, and thriving through the adversity. In fact, a study in the *Journal of Family Psychology* suggests that a higher sense of enduring control predicted lower levels of psychological distress and increases in control over time predicted decreases in depression and anxiety.[16]

There are several ways to take control. First, it's important to address mental health. Those facing adversity should

---

16 Courtney Pierce Keeton et al., "Sense of Control Predicts Depressive and Anxious Symptoms Across the Transition to Parenthood," *Journal of Family Psychology* 22, no. 2 (2008): 212-221.

talk to friends, neighbors, relatives, or a counselor about the trauma. Being open, honest, and vulnerable helps a survivor face adversity instead of burying it. They should also stay active. They should take part in movement when possible, which releases endorphins and can make them feel good. Survivors should try to get back to the routines they had when they were feeling their best. Routine can help them feel grounded and safe. By adding some controllable variables to our lives, we can empower ourselves to feel better sooner.

In my case, after floundering for a week adjusting to my terminal diagnosis, I finally found the courage to gain some control. The time had come to Google my fate. The average lifespan of someone diagnosed with stage four or metastatic breast cancer is two-and-a-half years. The five-year survivability is around 22 percent, and the ten-year survivability is between 1 and 4 percent.[17] I was one year into my MBA, I had a good job, a condominium in DC, great friends, and a busy social life, but my entire future passed in front of me. *What am I supposed to do now?*

Until this point in my life, almost everything I did was in preparation for something else. I was working on a second master's degree so I could gain traction in my career and grow my responsibility at work. I was trying to date in the difficult pool of singles as a thirty-something in Washington, DC, racing against that impending biological clock. I was serving my country part-time in the Army Reserves, preparing for my fourth rural health mission in five years. Everything I did was in preparation for the tomorrow, whenever and wherever that was. Almost none of my time was focused

---

[17] "Cancer Facts and Figures 2020," American Cancer Society, accessed August 29, 2020.

on present-day happiness, on the simple joys of living, or on the daily moments that could create true bliss.

In the years that have passed since that initial month, I've grown more than I've ever expected. I've outlived my prognosis. I've taken a hold of my treatment plan and faced things I've never thought possible. I've had over sixty-five rounds of chemotherapy, nineteen rounds of radiation, two surgeries, and four lymph nodes removed. But even more poignant, I've also added an extraordinary amount of purpose and meaning to my life. I've gained a new, special appreciation for the present. I've learned strategies to take control of what I can and relinquish guilt and responsibility for that which I can't.

I've even become thankful for my illness, for the perspective and enlightenment it's given me. I've built a community of survivors who have thrived in the face of adversity: from those involved in traumatic accidents, to life-changing diagnoses, to ongoing uncertainty that would, and should, demoralize someone completely. Each of these people, however, have instead looked at the face of their adversity as a challenge, even as a conquest to be had, and have asked themselves, "What am I going to do about this?"

Nancy was yearning for some control after her accident. She wasn't satisfied with her prognosis. Despite already beating the odds, she set out to do everything in her power to regain her abilities. She even pulled in the big guns. Nancy's daughter, a research scientist, was eager to help her create a plan that could potentially improve Nancy's odds of running, biking, and swimming again. So she started to send her journal articles, books, and studies that showed anything related to traumatic brain injuries and improved outcomes. Nancy dove into the research. She read twelve books on severe traumatic brain injuries and learned about miracle recoveries that others simply couldn't believe. She started to teach herself everything she could on brain recovery, and soon became an expert. Just because her therapists had thought she'd reached her peak didn't mean she had to accept that fate.

So Nancy started training. She worked for ten hours a day, seven days a week. After the first week, she was exhausted. This was the hardest thing she'd ever done. "This is harder than training for an Ironman," she thought. But every day, Nancy worked on her therapy. She had physical therapy and exercises, occupational therapy, and mental therapy. She worked on her physical health via exercises, her cognitive functioning using puzzles, and her emotional health with a therapist. She treated every bit of it like she was training for a race, and she was destined to come out on top.

Slowly, Nancy started improving. She started acupuncture for nerve health and found that sitting in a hypobaric oxygen chamber could help heal the brain. Week by week, she started to improve. At first, she'd walk to the end of the driveway. Then, she'd be able to walk down the street. Soon enough, Nancy was able to walk without a cane. But even with the physical progress, the one thing that wouldn't improve was her vision. Nancy had been experiencing terrible double vision. Her right and left eye were pointed in different directions because of her brain damage. "The doctors said it really wasn't treatable," she shared. So, Nancy took to her research.

It turns out, the phenomenon is called nonconvergence and it is hard to treat. Nevertheless, Nancy was determined. She found a specialist who treated nonconvergence, and he told her the treatment required daily work to rebuild the muscles in her eyes. His words were music to her ears. Nancy relished in the ability to put in the effort to make a difference, to have some control over her outcome. So she persevered. Every day she completed exercises for her eyes, in addition to her cognitive and physical exercises. Within a few months, Nancy had achieved perfect alignment. Her vision was completely restored.

Nancy isn't back to 100 percent physically; however, in only one year after her accident, she's already running, swimming, and biking. Her family once had very little hope that she'd ever recover; instead, she's thriving. In September, she and Adam performed their mother-son hip-hop number for the over two hundred guests at Adam's wedding. She had done it.

When I asked Nancy how she felt about her accident, she told me she'd never wish a traumatic brain injury on anyone and would give anything to have full functioning back, but she relishes in her ability to come as far as she has. She knows that not everyone could have made such a miraculous comeback. Her utter determination and dedication to having some control over her outcome has helped her overcome seemingly insurmountable odds.

Although Nancy and I have very different circumstances, we were both committed to controlling the variables that we could. In addition, we released worry about that which we couldn't. When facing any adversity, it's important to understand the difference. Empower yourself with what is known and what you can do to better yourself, but limit worry of things beyond your control. It's a fine line, but one that, once drawn, will help harness resilience at any point in your life.

CHAPTER 3

DEALING WITH BLAME

My friend, Dallas, was about to spend an epic Memorial Day weekend in Ocean City, Maryland. He was ready to party and live it up. Two days into his vacation, he made a split-second decision that changed his life and left him bound to a wheelchair forever.

In 2016, Dallas had excitedly ventured on a road trip to the beach city with a group of friends for a raucous weekend of fun. Just a few weeks before his twenty-seventh birthday, the scene was set for a great time. Dallas and his dozen or more friends rented a bougie house for the weekend. He knew gobs of people would be crowding the beach town for a weekend of fun. A true extrovert, Dallas was thrilled at the thought of meeting people and partying with the masses.

It's impossible to explain Dallas' vibrancy. I'd known him for a couple of years through mutual friends in Washington, DC. He's the kind of guy who you like immediately. His devilish smile and teasing personality make you both laugh and blush at the same time. Dallas is the life of the party. You can count on him to always be up for a good time. If Dallas came to an event, the party just seemed to thrive. Not only was he easy to talk to, but he was one of the best dancers I'd ever met. In DC, when we were out at the bars and there was space for dancing, Dallas would certainly be out there grooving.

I remember when Dallas told me that he went to college at Virginia Military Institute, which is a renowned military college known for exceedingly tough standards and a strict cadet experience. I could barely imagine someone as spirited as Dallas beholden to strict rules and regulations. But I somehow knew he thrived there. He even joined the college's division one diving program despite never having done it before. He's the kind of person who can make his way in just about any situation.

Most noticeably, Dallas was a people person. On Memorial Day weekend in 2016, he was ecstatic to be in Ocean City, one of the busiest beach towns in America. "I was just living life, living large," he said. Ocean City was the perfect opportunity to let loose. He had a new girlfriend, and she had joined him and his group of friends for a beach escape. They had planned a weekend that included restaurants, lounging on the beach, and, of course, the rowdy Ocean City bars. On the top of their list was one of the most notorious bars in Ocean City, Seacrets. During the summer, thousands of young people flock to this distillery slash bar slash beach party that sits right on the water. Seacrets even has its own beach and in-water seating for dining and boozing. If you wanted to party, and I mean *really party*, in Ocean City, this was your spot.

On the Sunday before Memorial Day, Dallas and his friends woke up after a late night and decided they'd continue their partying from the evening before. "The day before, we'd tried to get into Seacrets. We'd stood in line for four hours and still didn't make it in because it was so busy. So, this time, we were determined to get there early and find a spot."

Despite it being early in the day, the place was wild. People were everywhere. A few hours into the day, Dallas set out for the bathroom. Upon his return, his friends were nowhere to be found. Dallas looked around in frustration. The bar was enormous, and there were sweaty, drunk people everywhere. Dallas started to search around the bar, his efforts feeling futile after what felt like hours.

Eventually, he found himself outside, arguing with a bouncer about the whereabouts of his friends. "He had gotten upset with me for something, basically thinking I was acting smart." Despite his best efforts, Dallas wasn't able to convince the bouncer to let him back into the bar. "It was so frustrating, because my phone had gotten ruined the day before, so I realized I had no way of telling anyone where I was," he said, "So then, all I'm thinking now is, how do I get back in?"

Dallas had no phone, no car, and no way to get back to his house. He also had no way to get back into the bar. Frustrated, he started walking around the building trying to conjure up a plan. Eventually, he reached the back of the bar and found a nearby beach. Straining, he noticed that across the way, he could see the back entrance to Seacrets. Dallas wasn't deterred after seeing that it was roped off far into the water. If he could simply dive into the water and swim around the ropes, he could sneak up to the Seacrets private beach. This could be his way back in!

Looking around, Dallas noticed a dock jutting out into the water. He made his way over. At the end of the dock, he could just see the beach at Seacrets. Dallas thought for a minute. He was a collegiate diver, anyway, so, of course, he could navigate these waters without trouble. Dallas noticed a boat cruising nearby, but it was moving slowly, and it wasn't close enough to be dangerous. He also noticed two girls who were sitting and chatting on the dock, enjoying the sunshine and warm weather.

Dallas knew he could do this, despite his alcohol consumption that day and the unknown waters. He had to get back to his friends. So Dallas dove headfirst into the water. And then, everything went black.

The next day, Dallas woke up in a hospital. He could barely breathe. He felt large, obstructing tubes coming out of his mouth. His parents were standing in the room looking down at him with worried expressions. Dallas looked around, panicking, and tried to feel for his body. He could feel his face, blink his eyes, and move his mouth. But then he tried to reach for his family. In horror, he realized his arm wouldn't move. In that moment, Dallas realized he had lost all feeling below his face.

Dallas inadvertently dove into a very shallow part of the waterway and, upon entry, had broken his neck. He immediately lost consciousness. Dallas is still alive today because the two girls at the end of the pier immediately ran for help after they witnessed him dive and then surface face down and motionless. Even more serendipitous, the boat that was cruising nearby just happened to have one of Dallas' friend aboard. She, it turns out, is a nurse. After seeing the chaos, they immediately boated over to the scene. Within minutes, they'd coordinated a medivac to transport Dallas to the emergency room. Without this quick response, Dallas would have most certainly died. Even more fortuitous, Dallas' friend got in contact with his friends and, therefore, his family, almost immediately. Otherwise, no one would have known where he had disappeared to that day.

Dallas spent the next few weeks at a trauma hospital near Baltimore, Maryland. His doctors told him he was paralyzed, his life of partying and dancing was likely over, and he'd probably never walk again. A month later, Dallas transferred to a rehabilitation hospital in Atlanta where he'd stay for several months trying to regain any strength in his arms and legs.

The next few months were extremely trying for Dallas. He had lost all ability to function below the neck, including having control over his bowels. For the next month, he managed depressing thoughts. He wondered what his life would become without the use of his extremities. He imagined a life without dancing or traveling. He was devastated.

However, Dallas' therapists never gave up on him. He realized how important his efforts were in aiding recovery. Despite the initial diagnosis, Dallas started working to move various parts of his body. Each day, he got a little better at sensing movement. By making adjustments and staying on top of his therapy, he started to gain ability in his legs and right arm, which gave him a glimmer of hope.

Eventually, Dallas left the rehab hospital. Despite being in a wheelchair, he's not wheelchair bound. "I'm not a paraplegic because I experience paralysis in my upper body as well as my lower body. A paraplegic is only paralyzed in the lower body," he shared. "Technically, I am what is called an incomplete quadriplegic. You can also use the word Tetraplegia, as it's the more formal way to say quadriplegia. The reason it's incomplete is because my spinal cord wasn't completely severed. Although I'm weak and paralyzed, I can move different parts of my legs or arms, but every incomplete injury is different. I am just extremely lucky for the movement I was able to regain."

It's been four years since his accident, and whatever his diagnosis, he's thriving. He's regained function in several areas of his body, which is far more than initially predicted. He can stand on his own and use his right hand. "This is really what allows me to live such an independent life," he shared. His life has increased in difficulty tenfold and includes daily struggles such as navigating bathrooms, stairs, and wheelchair-inaccessible places. Despite this, Dallas' spirit has never wavered. "Being around people still lights me up," he shared. He's the same, vibrant human I met years ago, the same one who danced at every party. Now, he just dances a little differently.

Dallas has a unique mindset. He's thriving because he's determined to live a full and purposeful life despite his inabilities. He maintains the same spirit and vibrancy he's always had. Dallas has committed himself to having experiences. Since his illness, he's traveled all over the world. From Greece to Spain to Carnival in Brazil, if there's an experience to be had, Dallas is all over it. His will to live and determination to thrive is nothing short of inspiring.

Yet, like some other Thrivers, Dallas lives with some self-blame and regret. If only Dallas hadn't had alcohol that day, if only he hadn't gotten into an argument with the bouncer, if only he hadn't gone to Ocean City, if only he hadn't jumped off that pier, would he be dancing without a wheelchair today? For the first year of Dallas' recovery, he spent nights awake wondering what his life would be like if he had made just one different decision that day. He wonders what people think about his accident and subsequent disability. Is he forever to blame because he was the one who jumped into the water, he had been drinking, and he had been unrelenting in his determination to get back to his friends? Like Dallas, I've thought a lot about blame and how it can undermine our wellbeing and resilience. Those of us facing adversity can easily transition from "why me" to "of course this would happen to me." This level of ownership over injury, accident, or illness is generally counterproductive and can have a detrimental effect on our mindset, as well as our health. In fact, a research study in the *Journal of Social and Clinical Society* suggested that those with spinal cord injuries who blame themselves for their injury coped more poorly than those who attributed blame externally.[18]

Here's where we need to relinquish control: worrying about past experiences or thinking about the "what if" is an exercise in futility. If there's ever an opportunity to change your mindset, banishing self-blame should be your very first exercise. Blaming ourselves for past experiences or mistakes undermines both our mental and our physical health. It's linked to depression, guilt, shame, and even increased cortisol production, which creates an inflammatory response in our bodies and sends our stress level skyrocketing.[19]

I've had to face a lot of blame about my illnesses over the years. My first serious illness—the spinal tumor—was a diagnosis I practically celebrated. The tumor was treatable, I'd recover fully, get my pain-free life back, and nothing was my fault. Everyone was sympathetic to my pain, and not one

---

[18] Francisco Pagnini, Katherine Bercovitz, and Ellen Langer, "Perceived Control and Mindfulness: Implications for Clinical Practice," *Journal of Psychotherapy Integration* 26, no. 2 (February 2016): 91-102.

[19] George M. Slavich and Michael R. Irwin, "From Stress to Inflammation and Major Depressive Disorder: A Social Signal Transduction Theory of Depression," *Psychological Bulletin* 140, no. 3 (January 2014): 774-815.

person blamed me for my illness. I received a tremendous amount of support, love, and care.

At another time in my life, I was concerned about another illness. This time, I wasn't so sure I wasn't at least partly to blame.

During one of my summer breaks from college, I'd gotten a job as a dental assistant at an office in my hometown. I was still interested in medicine and wanted to see if a life in dentistry or orthodontia was in my future. I was excited for my first day. I arrived fifteen minutes early, which is uncharacteristic for a procrastinator like me. I spent the first few hours getting the lay of the land, learning the tools, the dental molds, and the sterilizing equipment. Patients started to trickle in. I'd greet them and help them get set up for their appointment with various sheaths and protective coverings.

Toward the end of the day, however, the dentist asked if I'd help with a procedure. "Yes!" I exclaimed, excitedly. The time had come to get in on the action. Before we went into the procedural room, the dentist briefed me. He was performing an extraction. All I had to do was stand on the other side of the patient and hand the dentist his tools. I nodded in agreement.

We entered the room and I exchanged pleasantries with the patient. The doctor started the procedure immediately. "Sickle probe," he said. I handed him the tool with a long handle with a sharp hook on the end. The dentist started to poke around the patient's mouth, and I looked in with fascination. Then, the world went blank.

I awoke a few minutes later to the doctor holding what I would learn later were smelling salts at my nose. I was flat on my back at the foot of the patient chair, bewildered by what had just transpired. "You passed out," the doctor told me. "You fell onto the patients' lap, and then rolled down his legs to the floor." I looked up at the patient in sheer horror. I collected myself and hurried to the break room. I was asked to not work with patients for the rest of my summer job. I only lasted one more week, mortified by the altercation that had transpired, the one that everyone in the office seemed unwilling to forget.

For the next few years, I had several incidents of fainting, sometimes at the sight of blood, sometimes after getting up too quickly. Finally, in graduate school, we were testing our own blood sugar and I returned a high result. I was embarrassed. I was of "normal" weight and exercised regularly, but I was showing signs of impaired fasting glucose, which is the first indication of type 2 diabetes. In my mind, I had brought this on myself.

As a child and teen, I struggled with consistently making poor diet choices, which included frequent sodas and daily candy. I never ate vegetables. I only liked white bread. At this point, I had grown significantly and was making much better food choices as well as studying to become a Registered Dietitian, but I was always concerned that my poor diet set me up for health issues as an adult. My history embarrassed me. I was determined not to share my test results with anyone for fear they'd blame or judge me for my misfortune.

Many illnesses are in that grey area, which are potentially caused by lifestyle choices, family genes, or simply by chance. Many people have dealt with these maladies at one time in their life and have probably received some unsolicited advice on how to rectify their illnesses. It's not uncommon to feel a variety of emotions when receiving unsolicited advice for an illness or injury you've endured: hurt, disappointment, indignation, or even anger. But blaming other people for their illnesses can make us feel better about ourselves. It might even make us feel like we're not vulnerable to a similar fate. If someone gets coronary artery disease, it's easy to say, "I eat a lot of fruits and vegetables, so that's not going to happen to me." Somehow, qualifying their illness feels right in the moment. The resulting feeling for the other person is blame for their misfortune.

The truth is that blaming others helps no one. Whether obesity, mental illness, fibromyalgia, diabetes, or a traumatic accident, luck plays into each person's fate as much as their choices. But as humans, we feel judgment toward other people because we want to close the gap of information. We're naturally curious. We want to feel disconnected personally from another person's adversity. We think, *That can't happen to me.*

However, if we spent more time supporting each other by listening and observing without judgment, we'd be able to develop a healthy environment for all. When you judge someone, it affects you more than the other person. It says more about you than the other person. You convey how you perceive the world. It shows the preconceptions your mind has. Instead of judgment, observe and be curious. Seek more information. Expand the gap between observation and conclusion.[20]

I've talked to Dallas about how blame has affected his relationship with others. "You know, I spent a fair amount of time feeling depressed about what happened that day," he shared, "And when I'm around other people, it was easier for me to joke about my illness and my situation than

---

20 Prakar Verma, "How to Develop a Non-judgmental Attitude to Live More Peacefully," *The Startup* (blog), September 27, 2018.

talk seriously. It made other people more comfortable to be around me." Dallas may joke about his accident or his life in a wheelchair, but he doesn't joke about blame. He knows that his choice to jump headfirst into the water that day changed his life forever, and if he had made one different choice, he may not be in a wheelchair right now. Dallas also realizes that harboring blame is simply pointless.

"It is what it is," he says. "It's not even worth wishing I could go back. All I can do now is the best I can with my situation and pay it forward for others who may have to deal with what I have to deal with now." Instead of wallowing in blame, Dallas has dedicated himself to the United Spinal Cord Association, where he even serves as the Washington, DC chapter Fundraising Committee Chair. He was selected to represent their chapter at the National conference in the last three National Leadership Conferences, spreading hope and encouragement to others with spinal cord injuries. Although his accident may have changed his life, he relishes in the opportunities he has now to motivate others with his inspirational story. "I honestly wouldn't change how my life turned out," he said.

It turned out that my brush with pre-diabetes was short-lived. However, it did motivate me to make significant changes in the food I ate, and it got me thinking about how we manage blame in our lives. While I never blamed myself for my spinal tumor, I've experienced some level of guilt about my breast cancer. What, if anything, did I do to cause this cancer to form so aggressively considering my lack of family history of cancer? It seemed obvious that something in my environment triggered my illness, so what did I do wrong? For months, I thought back to the food I ate and the potential environments I'd been exposed to. Desperate to understand, many people joined in on the wonderment, even my own family. "Why do you think this happened?" someone would ask. I'd simply shake my head.

After I got through my first few rounds of chemo and lost all my hair and part of my dignity, I decided I was never going to blame myself again for my illness. It simply wasn't worth it. I'd endured some of the harshest treatments a person could manage. Despite the reason for its onset, I was dealt a merciless hand in life. At this point, however, I had a choice. I could either keep searching for the reason this happened to me, or I could relinquish the blame, and hone in on how I could come out on top.

I chose the latter.

CHAPTER 4

POST-TRAUMATIC GROWTH

After my spinal tumor and subsequent surgery, I thought I was on the clear road to recovery. I could not have been more wrong.

I'd finished college, played my final softball game, and started my journey toward my dream of becoming a sports dietitian. I was in my second year of graduate school, and I started to feel alternating aching and sharp pain in my neck. "No way," I thought, "this can't be happening again."

I had an apartment and a job in Pennsylvania, where I went to school, but I immediately abandoned it. I had the summer off before my final year of school, and I needed to figure out what was wrong. I moved back in with my parents and immediately got an appointment to see my doctors at Johns Hopkins. Right away, we started with a battery of tests. Had my tumor returned? Was it the brain malformation? Was it time for the decompression surgery to relieve the pressure on my brain?

After a few inconclusive tests, we were back to the drawing board. My doctors weren't totally sure what was wrong. They could see there was no tumor regrowth and my brain malformation hadn't exacerbated, so it was likely not the source of the problem. In a last-ditch effort, my neurosurgeon sent me to get a discogram. This somewhat unusual test was meant to determine whether my cervical disc was damaged and leaking fluid. He thought the method they used to stabilize my spine during my tumor surgery could have failed and may have been starting to crush my disc. This kind of compression could be very painful and would require another surgery to make things right again.

I went in for the discogram thinking this would be a simple procedure. But this test was anything but normal. Assuming I'd be in twilight or some state of unconsciousness, I certainly wasn't prepared for the test. As soon as I arrived, I asked the radiologist who was performing the test, "Will I feel anything during this test?"

"Oh yes! That's the whole point."

As it turns out, a discogram is an invasive procedure that relies on your feedback to determine the structural integrity of your spinal discs. While viewing an x-ray monitor, the doctor inserts the hollow needle through your skin directly into your spine, to the center of the disc space, while he or she looks on. Once the needle is in place, a dye is injected into the disc that shows up white on the x-rays. The discogram works in two ways—both to view the disc and to find the source of pain. The doctor injects the dye into the disc space to try to recreate the pain. If you feel pain, then that disc is the likely source of your pain.

Sure enough, a few minutes into my test, I was screeching with pain. My C 4-5 disc was completely damaged, leaking fluid, and needed to be removed.

After the trauma of the discogram, my doctor called me with the news. Clearly, I had disc damage. The good news is that with surgery, they could remove the disc and add a plate and two screws that could, instead, support my spinal column. Compared to my tumor surgery, it was a relatively short surgery and wouldn't require a long recovery. In fact, my surgeon could make an incision in the front of my neck instead of the back, resulting in much less damage to my muscular tissue.

I was relieved. We'd found the source of the pain and I could simply schedule my surgery. Unfortunately, getting there wasn't quite so easy.

I was two years into my graduate program and, thus, had been kicked off of my parent's insurance. I had enrolled in the health insurance provided by my school. Immediately, as we began the pre-authorization to prepare for surgery, my insurance balked. This issue, they quipped, was due to my tumor surgery. The preexisting condition would render me ineligible for this second surgery. I could either pay the $75,000 for my surgery or I'd be out of luck.

We fought for months as I moved back to Pennsylvania to finish my last year of school. To avoid the pain, I took daily oxycodone, which caused me to become dependent on the narcotic drug. I lived in a state of mild confusion every day, the narcotic taking a toll on my mental health. The pain had gotten so severe that I couldn't live without it. I remember trying to go back to work and class and having dizziness that left me incapacitated. But if I stopped taking the medications, I was in excruciating pain. It seemed as if there was no way out.

Eventually, six months after my discogram, we went ahead with the surgery. I agreed upon a payment plan with the hospital to cover the bills. Even though I was only making about $15,000 a year working part-time supporting myself through graduate school, I simply couldn't live in pain any longer.

The surgery, a discectomy and spinal fusion, was a fantastic success. The surgeons were able to make a minor incision, remove my damaged disc, and screw a titanium plate into my spinal column. Just a few days after returning home from my surgery, I was up and walking. I went back to school only a couple of weeks later. Most importantly, I was pain-free again.

I paid my monthly payment to the hospital for more than a year, sacrificing just about all frivolous purchases, as I continued to fight with my insurance. I moved out of my apartment in Pennsylvania and back into my parents' house. I corralled my last few classes into one day per week so I could drive eight hours round trip to avoid paying rent. How could this preexisting clause really be a rule? Neither of these conditions was my fault. Was I not allowed to have subsequent care for my neck for the rest of my life? Luckily, my surgeon was on my side. He worked diligently, writing multiple letters to my insurance company assuring them that my two surgeries, although occurring at the exact same cervical level, were not related. As he stated, the discectomy and subsequent spinal fusion was an anomaly, and a simple coincidence that it happened to be located in the same spot as my tumor once was. I know it was a farce, but I also didn't care. It wasn't fair in either situation.

I had a rare spinal tumor and instability that had crushed my disc only five years later, which wasn't my fault. Was I supposed to live in pain forever because of it?

Eventually, the insurance company complied. Not only did they pay for my surgery, but they paid me back the monthly payments I'd made to the hospital. I think they felt sorry for me, or maybe someone realized the injustice of the preexisting clause. Or maybe my doctor was particularly adept at fudging the truth. Whatever it was, I was overjoyed. It had been a year-and-a-half process, from the authorization of the surgery to the payment, to a month-long weening off of narcotics, but I was completely pain-free and it was worth it.

At this point in my life, I was starting to experience more adversity, a contrast to what I'd faced growing up. After my second spinal surgery and the subsequent complications with insurance and payment, I could feel my skin thickening. For some reason, my health experiences were helping me improve my mental wellbeing in a very real way. In thinking about this, I discovered a term that started to help me understand how adversity can lead to rebounding, an improved sense of gratitude, an improved outlook, or overall resilience.

This learning, called post-traumatic growth, involves "life-changing" psychological shifts in thinking and relates to the world around you. The whole process is somewhat existential, as the person experiencing it seems to be able to see the world differently after trauma or adversity. After my second surgery, I was starting to truly understand that there would be elements of my life that I couldn't control, and that life could be hard and unfair, and that was okay. I was empowered by it. Each time adversity hit, I'd feel proud to have been able to tackle the obstacle, and it built me up just a little bit more.

The term "post-traumatic growth" was coined in the mid-1990s by Richard Tedeschi and Lawrence Calhoun, who are both psychologists. "People develop new understandings of themselves, the world they live in, how to relate to other people, the kind of future they might have, and a better understanding of how to live life," says Tedeschi.[21]

Post-traumatic growth, however, is not the same as inherent resilience. "Post-traumatic growth is sometimes considered synonymous with resilience because becoming more resilient as a result of a struggle with trauma can be an example of PTG. But PTG is different from resilience," says Kanako Taku, PhD, associate professor of psychology at Oakland University, who has both researched PTG and experienced it as a survivor of the 1995 Kobe earthquake in Japan. "Resiliency is the personal attribute or ability to bounce back," he says, "PTG, on the other hand, refers to what can happen when someone who has difficulty bouncing back experiences a traumatic event that challenges his or her core beliefs, endures psychological struggle, and then ultimately finds a sense of personal growth." In other words, post-traumatic growth can help build resilience. It's a testament that resilience can be earned and learned, and isn't something we're all born with or without.[22]

A key indicator of this phenomenon is how the individual sees themselves after trauma. Those who experience post-traumatic growth begin to see themselves stronger as a result of their healing. They shift the view of the trauma away from a sickness or illness that has happened to them, and instead, the trauma becomes an impact. Instead of "what is wrong with me," the thought becomes, "what has happened to me."[23]

---

21 Richard G. Tedeschi and Lawrence G. Calhoun, "Posttraumatic Growth: Conceptual Foundations and Empirical Evidence," *Psychological Inquiry* 15, no. 1 (2004): 1-18.
22 Ibid.
23 Ibid.

Between 30 to 70 percent of individuals who experienced trauma also report positive change and growth coming out of the traumatic experience. Although not many people would wish for trauma to occur, many do see the true value of their experience. They're stronger because of it.[24]

Kate, my friend of over fifteen years, is a true warrior. She has experienced post-traumatic growth many times over. I've known her since we started graduate school together. Both of us have a deep passion for nutrition and the human body. I immediately liked Kate. She had a soft, soothing way about her, and she was very open. I learned that she had a son at a young age and had moved all around the country in hopes of a good life for her and her son. Her passion for nutrition brought her back to her hometown of Scranton, Pennsylvania to pursue a master's degree in nutrition. As she and I got closer, I started to learn more about her life and the struggles she'd endured already at such a young age.

When Kate was a teenager, she felt tired all the time. Many people in her life chalked it up to depression or assumed she was struggling with an underlying mental illness. But Kate was trying hard to live life as normally as possible. She even ran on the cross-country team at her high school. Unfortunately, after she ran, she always felt somewhat ill. She was slow to recover, and she remembers hearing her heartbeat very loudly. She didn't know if that was normal for all people, so she simply kept it to herself.

When Kate turned seventeen, she unexpectedly got pregnant. In preparation for her delivery, she had a full workup with an obstetrician. Her doctors put her on a new medicine,

---

[24] Stephen Joseph, "What Doesn't Kill Us," *The Psychologist* 25 (November 2012): 816-819.

which was sometimes given to teen mothers to prevent preterm labor. Kate remembers having strange feelings in her heart shortly thereafter. "I was having palpitations, but the doctors kept telling me that was normal for the medication," she shared. Luckily, Kate's pregnancy and delivery went fine, and within a few months, she had a healthy baby boy.

When her son was just a few months old, however, Kate couldn't ignore the nagging sensation. "I just had this intuitive sense that there was something wrong," she said, "I had an irritating cough that wouldn't go away. So, I went to my family doctor and he just put me off with an antibiotics prescription." Kate thinks this happens a lot with young, otherwise healthy women. "They get brushed off, like, nothing is wrong with you. You're just depressed and tired because you just had a baby."

Despite her age, Kate had the emotional maturity not to accept no for an answer. Looking back, she's proud of herself. "I pushed hard to get an answer; I knew something was wrong," she said. Finally, she got some answers.

Kate was at another postpartum appointment, and, to her surprise, her doctor was out of the office. Luckily, Kate was able to see his colleague. Upon completing her normal exam, the new doctor turned to Kate. "Did you know you have a heart murmur?"

Kate was floored. She'd been to the doctor multiple times during her pregnancy, many of which she'd been checked with a stethoscope.

But Kate's mom was there with her. "I have a heart murmur too, and it's benign. Yours probably is too."

Luckily, Kate's new doctor wanted to be cautious. "Let's send you to a cardiologist and get you an echocardiogram." This decision saved her life.

The echocardiogram showed that Kate had a disease of her heart valves. When she went to the cardiologist, she was the youngest person in the waiting room by decades. She didn't know what to expect. And then, her doctor shared the insane news that rocked her world. "You're going to need at least two open heart surgeries in your life. One will have to be pretty soon. I can't actually believe you went through labor, knowing how much strain that put on your heart. Unfortunately, you won't be able to have any more children."

Kate was living with a ticking time bomb in her chest. She didn't know anyone else her age who had to deal with heart disease. Suddenly, she was keenly aware of her health, never knowing when the bomb would go off. In fact, the life expectancy of someone with heart valve disease is significantly less than someone with a healthy heart.[25]

For Kate, this new diagnosis brought about a sense of urgency she hadn't had before. "I've got to hurry up and live my life because I don't know how long I have," she shared. Her mom suggested she stay at home and get a low-paying job to help pay the bills and support her child, but with a greater sense of uncertainty, Kate went after her goals instead. She packed up her son and moved to the West Coast, realizing her dreams of going away to college on her own. "I developed that attitude early; if I wanted to do something, I was going to do it. Right now."

Kate had several good years. She finished college and eventually moved back to complete a master's degree in nutrition, where she and I met. At the same time, I was learning

---

25 "Life Expectancy after Aortic Valve Replacement," Relias Media, accessed June 12, 2020.

about my disc disease, Kate was getting the news that it was time for her open heart surgery.

At this point, Kate was getting out of breath from the simplest of chores. She'd be folding laundry and could barely catch her breath. Sure enough, after a few tests, her cardiologist told her that her valves were in rough shape. One was regurgitating blood, so the blood was flowing backward. There simply wasn't enough oxygenating blood flowing through her body. The other valve had stenosis or narrowing of the vessel. So Kate went to see a surgeon in Philadelphia. Immediately, he confirmed it. "This is urgent. You're in heart failure right now."

At twenty-nine years old, Kate had surgery right away. She had two diseased valves, but the surgeons could only replace one during the procedure. They replaced her aortic valve with an animal valve with the hope it would last for ten to fifteen years. All Kate could do is hope and pray the surgery would take and give her many more years with her son. She also knew she'd have to have surgery again, this time to replace both valves. Regardless, her attitude changed immediately. "I have to live, if not for myself, for him," she shared.

Kate's recovery was not easy. She experienced a lot of pain. It took more than a year for her to get back to feeling like herself again. She knew she'd have to have another surgery at some point, but she felt somehow empowered. Knowing she'd have more trauma to endure made it easier to manage somehow. "I just always had it in my head that I'd have to deal with this again, an even bigger surgery, at some point. But I was prepared."

Those of us who have experienced a traumatic event or illness understand the range of emotions you can encounter. I certainly know I experienced a lot of the "why me?" when I was first diagnosed with cancer. However, many people thrive not despite their illness or trauma, but because of it. Tedeschi and Calhoun noted that 90 percent of traumatic event survivors reported at least one positive change as a result of trauma. In fact, research has suggested that more victims experience growth than develop psychiatric disorders.[26]

It's important to understand that these people grow because they've acknowledged their trauma; they haven't buried it. People who have suffered from trauma can go through a period of obsessing about or wallowing in the pain of their experience, and this is incredibly common. Ignoring or avoiding thoughts about the emotional fallout of a tragedy can be equally as harmful to long-term growth.[27]

Psychologist Dr. David Feldman says, "Trauma survivors who experience PTG acknowledge their own sadness, suffering, anger, and grief, and are realistic about what happened to them," adding that they then ask the question, "How can I build the best future possible?"[28]

The measurement of post-traumatic growth is categorized into five major domains: greater appreciation of life, more intimate relationships with others, greater personal strength, recognition of new possibilities in life, and spiritual or religious growth. Some experts believe post-traumatic growth is actually a coping mechanism to help survivors overcome their shattered worldview and sense of vulnerability. It may be an adaptive tool for revising the narrative of one's life and simply returning to equilibrium.[29]

---

[26] Lorna Collier, "Growth after Trauma," *Monitor on Psychology* 47, no. 10 (November 2016): 48.
[27] Stephen Joseph, ibid.
[28] Ibid.
[29] Ginny Graves, "Is There an Upside to Tragedy," *Oprah* (blog), July 2015.

After I recovered from my second spinal surgery, something in me had changed significantly. I'd experienced two major surgeries, each with their own issues, from skeptical doctors to a preexisting clause mishap. I was a few months away from finishing my master's degree, and I felt like my ability to overcome these two events helped prepare me for the real world. I'd experienced real, overwhelming pain, a narcotics addiction, financial insecurity, and health uncertainty, all before I was twenty-five. When I started my first full-time job, rented my first apartment on my own, and started dealing with life's issues, they paled in comparison to my health struggles. I used my illnesses and adversity as a stool to prop myself up. If I could handle this, I could easily handle other things that life threw at me.

For Kate, she spent a lot of time thinking about why she had to deal with her rare and unusual life-altering heart condition. Her heart condition was not caused by anything she did, anything to do with her lifestyle, or anything she ate. A doctor once told her it was simply bad luck. "I think I had to give up any illusion of control," she shared. "Of course, I went through this period where I really wanted to know why this happened to me. I mean, nobody else in my family has had to endure this. But the truth is, there's really no explanation, and I've come to terms with that."

Only eleven years after her first surgery, Kate had to have open heart surgery to replace both of her heart valves. Both had finally failed. Her surgery lasted nine hours, and she experienced an unexpected complication. Some tissue from the previously implanted tissue valve had grown up and around the wall of her heart. The surgeons had to scrape it all away and off the heart wall, resulting in a lot of blood loss. They then had to replace her whole aortic root. Kate woke up very sick and ended up having a traumatic recovery, including several blood transfusions. She lost fifteen pounds in a week.

Kate was in the hospital for some time. Eventually, her doctors cleared her to return home. Two days after she returned home, she experienced a new complication. "It was like an earthquake went off in my body, inside my heart," she shared. Kate returned to the hospital, where her heart rate was over two hundred beats per minute. She was readmitted for five more days. Subsequently, Kate went through many ups and downs during her recovery, ranging from depression to complete fatigue.

Initially, she felt a euphoric sensation that she had survived and was alive, but she also felt like she had been run over by a truck. "I was weak and diminished, a shadow of my former self," she said. She couldn't walk her dog. She couldn't lift her arms to wash her hair. Her family had to hire a caregiver to take care of Kate's basic needs. She was demoralized.

Eventually, Kate started to recover. She started to be more transparent about her illness within her community. She started to be more open about her mindset with her doctor. He said, "You've been through a trauma. It's a controlled trauma, but it's a trauma." Kate started to take a more proactive approach to her recovery. She visited a pain management specialist who helped her ease the daily, crippling pain. She started physical therapy and working with a psychologist.

It took her more than fifteen months to get to a point where she felt like herself again. "I had to go through a process where I had to accept that I wasn't the same Kate as I was going into that surgery. I had to let go of that person." She released the idea that she could go back to the way things were. They were never going to be that way again. She had to accept her new normal.

Kate has experienced the pressure to do more with her life. Many Thrivers do. They feel like they have to do more things quicker because of the uncertainty their life holds. Kate, however, has realized that she doesn't need to do everything to get to happiness. "I can do amazing things. I can raise my kid. I can be there for him. I can be there for my husband. I can be there for my parents, siblings, my stepdaughter, and friends. I don't need to change the world. I'm at peace with that."

Many people have shared that Kate's strength has been inspiring to them, and she's the strongest person they know. While that puts pressure on Kate, she also knows that simply living through her trauma is an inspiration, and should be celebrated. "I never would have believed I was strong enough to get through these things. But I am truly stronger on the other side," she says. "And I'm a better healthcare practitioner because of it. I have better empathy; I understand trauma and adversity. I have better patience and can be totally present for them."

Although Kate would never choose her heart issue, she knows she's a stronger person because of it.

Many of you might be struggling to harness your resilience because you haven't experienced life-altering trauma, but know this: trauma comes in many forms. You don't need to be diagnosed with cancer, have multiple organ failures, or come close to death to grow your resilience. You can experience growth from any adversity. Practice on small things such as bad traffic, poor weather, and failed plans. Look for the good, the silver lining in each and every situation. Find ways to acknowledge your struggle and then consciously move forward. These micro-growths will start building your resilience muscles before you even need it.

PART 2

PRINCIPLES OF RESILIENCE

CHAPTER 5

DEFIANCE

My friend, Stephanie, is one of the most resilient, albeit defiant, people I've ever known. Tell her no and she'll show you what yes looks like. She's the kind of person you always want on your side, but you'd be better off never telling her what to do or how to live her life.

I've been friends with Stephanie for twenty-five years. We've been in each other's lives through all of the hurdles. We experienced adolescence, young love, trauma, separation, sadness, empathy, and celebrations together. I was the maid of honor at her wedding. She was one of the first people I called when I was diagnosed with cancer. She's my family.

Stephanie, however, had a different upbringing than me. My parents were involved with just about every sport I played, every activity, every lesson. They'd show up at tennis matches and hide in the bushes because I felt smothered by their attention. Stephanie's mom, on the other hand, passed away at a young age. Her father had a variety of jobs, including owning and managing property. He also worked as a gourmet French chef in various upscale restaurants in DC, returning home late at night. Stephanie's sisters were much older than her.

They moved out of the house when they turned eighteen, so Stephanie was left alone a lot. When Stephanie and I became friends, I was fourteen and she was thirteen. She was already the most independent person I'd ever met. Stephanie and I had a close relationship throughout high school. We pushed the boundaries of high school life just like many kids do—sneaking out, trying new things, drinking wine coolers. Stephanie made her own rules and wasn't a fan of the word "no." When we were together, I felt like the world was an endless possibility. I became more independent, nourished my free spirit, and started to define who I was. Stephanie was such a passionate advocate for herself, me, her friends, and her family. She made her own rules, and I've always admired her for it.

When Stephanie left for college at the age of seventeen, I knew she'd never come back. Right away, Stephanie created a new life for herself. She worked tirelessly throughout college, not only in her studies but also in various jobs during the school year and over the summer. Stephanie had to pay for college herself, and her dedication to leave school without loans was admirable. After college, a career in marketing and a handful of relationships took her to a variety of places, from southern Virginia to North Carolina, and eventually to Cincinnati. She came back here to go back to school to become a Registered Dietitian too. I like to think I influenced her decision to shift her career focus to health and nutrition. It's also brought us even closer together, despite not having lived in the same town for more than a decade.

Stephanie got married relatively young and had two children, a boy and a girl. She moved back to North Carolina when she got pregnant the third time. She had a normal, easy pregnancy, but I remember her due date coming and going and not hearing a word from her or her husband Ryan. I sent her a text a few days later, asking if everything was okay. I received a text back. "We're okay. It was a complicated delivery. I'll update you later." She was not normally so curt. I was immediately concerned.

Stephanie had delivered her third child, a beautiful boy named Benson, in October of 2017. During labor, Benson's heart rate was nonviable, and once delivered, he wasn't breathing. "He had a collapsed lung and brain damage from a severe brain injury due to a loss of oxygen and blood flow during delivery," Stephanie said. Benson was resuscitated, intubated, and placed in a hypothermic state to preserve his brain function. After several days and many tests, the doctors diagnosed him with Hypoxic Ischemic Encephalopathy (HIE). The doctors told Stephanie and her husband Ryan that his brain damage was so severe that there was a good chance Benson wouldn't live past two weeks.

Stephanie, having worked in clinical dietetics in various hospitals, had some insight about what would give Benson his best chance for survival. Shortly after birth, Stephanie and her husband sent Benson on a medical flight to Cincinnati Children's Hospital. The doctors there confirmed the extent of the brain damage. Benson was in the NICU for a little over a month and was sent home with little hopes of survival. In fact, his doctors hypothesized he wouldn't live to see his first birthday.

This damage to Benson's brain has led to several secondary diagnoses, such as cerebral palsy and epilepsy. He is legally blind, has a hearing impairment, and cannot safely swallow or clear his airway, requiring a feeding tube to be surgically placed into his stomach; called a G tube. Currently, Benson receives traditional therapies like PT, OT, Speech

Therapy, and Vision Education. But Benson's doctors have never been optimistic about his prognosis. "I've pushed them to be more aggressive in his treatment, to include things such as CBD oil, oxygen therapy, and stem cells, but not one of his doctors has provided us with any hope for Benson's brain development," she shared. Despite this, they've persevered. In fact, their apathy toward Benson's recovery has somehow fueled Stephanie. She's taken on full responsibility for Benson's health and uses the doctors more like consultants to his care plan. No one knows her son like she does, and no one knows what he's capable of.

It's this defiance, and her unwavering love and commitment to her family, that fuels Stephanie. I truly believe this is why her son is still alive two years later.

Some of the most powerful stories I've heard in life are those in which people have been told they can't do something. We're all motivated when we hear someone "proved *them* wrong," whomever the "them" is. We all get that twinge of defiance when told we can't do something. It fuels a little fire inside us.

I believe there's power in that struggle. When someone says they don't expect us to succeed, many people can be motivated by these "underdog expectations." Dr. Samir Nurmohamed, a researcher at the Wharton School of Business at the University of Pennsylvania, has researched this phenomenon and found that, by having naysayers in our lives, we can be motivated to far outperform ourselves otherwise. Dr. Nurmohamed surveyed 371 employees in a consumer-packaged-goods company, asking about the extent to which they were seen as an underdog by others. Seven weeks later, their supervisors evaluated their performance. He found that experiencing "underdog expectations" was a significant predictor of performance, even after controlling for employees' own expectations for success. In other words, people who believed that others did not expect them to be successful were more likely to receive higher performance evaluations from their supervisors.[30]

These results showed a positive correlational link between underdog expectations and work performance. But Dr. Nurmohamed wanted to see if randomly assigned feedback would make a difference in work performance as well. He conducted a follow-up experiment with 330 online workers, asking them to do a computer task that involved clicking on rapidly moving circles. They were told someone was observing their performance on the task. After participants completed a fifteen-second practice round, they received one of three messages—stating underdog expectations, high expectations, or neutral expectations—from the observer. Unbeknownst to them, the expectations were randomly assigned. Participants then performed the task, which was five minutes long and required a combination of effort and focus to do effectively. He found that those who experienced underdog expectations performed the best—above and beyond those who received high or neutral expectations.[31]

In short, there's marked value to being told you *can't*.

Like Stephanie, I've learned that having defiance helps to fuel my drive. When I started to look at colleges, I had a naive, singular focus. I wanted to go where I could be an athlete and excel at my sport. I applied only to colleges that had expressed interest in my athletic ability. In the fall of

---

30 Samir Nurmohame, "The Underdog Effect: When Low Expectations Increase Performance," *Academy of Management Journal* 63, no. 4 (August 24, 2020).
31 Ibid.

my senior year, I visited several schools to narrow down my choices: Bucknell, UNC Chapel Hill, Virginia Tech, Villanova, and James Madison University. However, my father had played lacrosse at the University of Delaware, so he convinced me to look at their softball program. I decided it'd be worth a day trip up to Wilmington.

I remember the drive to Delaware not because it was substantial by any means, but because this was one of the first trips I would make to talk to a division one coach about my abilities. I was nervous but also excited. I'd spent time the previous spring putting together a recruiting tape that showcased my abilities as a shortstop and hitter. I'd sent it to the coach a week earlier and couldn't wait to hear her feedback.

After the two-hour drive, my dad and I found the athletic department and made our way to the softball coach's office. Butterflies filled my stomach. Even though this school wasn't my top choice, I was excited to get feedback from a real college coach. Since she'd invited me on this trip after seeing my talent, I knew she'd welcome me to her school and team.

My dad and I sat down, and the coach joined us in a small room next to her office. She shook our hands and then looked at me straight in the eye. "Listen, I took this meeting because your Dad is an alumnus. But I watched your video. On a scale of 1 to 5, I think your skill level ranks about 2.5. I don't think you have the talent to play division one softball."

The meeting was over in less than ten minutes. I wasn't quite sure how to respond to the coach's comments. She wasn't mean; she was simply honest and direct. I wasn't good enough, not just to play on her team but to play for any division one program. My hopes of playing at the elite level were dashed in a matter of minutes. My heart dropped. I remember walking out of the building and bursting into tears, mortified that we'd made such an effort. My dad was stunned into silence, and we journeyed the two hours home brimming with confusion, frustration, and disappointment.

Luckily, other coaches saw some potential in my video—not all, but some—and I was asked to play for a couple of division one colleges. A few years later, I was the starting center fielder on JMU's division one softball team. During my first season, I took a look at our spring schedule and immediately noticed a familiar foe: The University of Delaware. Since Delaware was in our conference, each year we'd get to play a triple-header with the Blue Hens over the course of a weekend. I'd get to come face-to-face with that coach for three games in a row. I looked forward to it every year.

Each time, without fail, I had my best games of the season against Delaware. I hit doubles, triples, and home runs. I had diving catches and stolen bases. It didn't matter if I was in a slump during the season; I shined at the Delaware games. When it came to the conference awards, the Delaware coach raised her hand to vote for me as I was recognized as an all-conference standout for two years in a row.

I've often thought about those games and why I was able to play so well. What was it about that coach and my absolute resolve to play my best? I was so hurt by her brutal comments, and so determined to prove her wrong. Playing well against her was my only defense mechanism. I took the opportunity to showcase exactly what she could have had if she had signed me. *This is what a 2.5 looks like now.*

Why do underdogs seem to perform better in these kinds of situations? We all love the stories of *David and Goliath* and *The Tortoise and the Hare* because it's easy to root for the one you'll assume won't win. We find ourselves drawn to stories about big businesses like Microsoft that had an improbable start in a garage, or writers like J. K. Rowling who experienced poverty while writing about Harry Potter. Perhaps it's because we see ourselves in these stories, and they give us permission to dream big.

Those of us facing cancer or any other serious illness have an even bigger motivation to take a fighting stance. According to a study on attitudes and breast cancer, higher rates of recurrence-free survival were reported in patients who initially responded with attitudes of a "fighting spirit."[32] Another study showed that a five-year survival chance in breast cancer patients was improved significantly in those patients who had taken on a fighting attitude compared to a helpless or hopeless one. In addition, there was a significant chance of death after five years when the patient had adopted the latter attitudes.[33]

While attitude during illness is a very popular topic of discussion, it's not without its controversies. It's near impossible to assess someone's attitude all the time. Collecting this kind of data requires constant monitoring or 100 percent accurate self-reported data. While we may never know specifically how a fighting attitude impacts our ability to combat disease, we know it is beneficial to our outlook, environment, and sense of wellbeing. So it certainly can't hurt. It's one more variable we have that's totally within our control.

Thanks in part to Stephanie's utter determination, Benson has lived two years longer than anyone predicted. Stephanie

---

[32] D. V. Nelson et al., "Attitudes of Cancer: Psychometric Properties of Fighting Spirit and Denial," *Journal of Behavioral Medicine* 12, no. 4 (August 1989): 341-355.

[33] Mark Petticrew, Ruth Bell, and Duncan Hunter, "Influence of Psychological Coping on Survival and Recurrence in People with Cancer: Systematic Review," *BMJ* 325 (November 9, 2002).

and Ryan are fully committed to his care, and Stephanie's defiance continues to reign. She's so used to hearing "no he can't," that it doesn't even phase her anymore. Luckily, he's surpassed all expectations. His regular pediatricians are always blown away by Benson's resiliency and Stephanie's commitment to his care. They're also stunned at Benson's progress. Stephanie takes him to regular oxygen therapy. She has traveled to various spots in Latin America to get him stem cell treatments, which are not currently approved in the US. His brain is showing signs of development, and he's building new neuropathways. Despite all odds, he's showing growth and progress.

I think about Stephanie all the time. When we're able to catch up on the phone, our conversations easily last an hour and a half. She's always with Benson because he requires twenty-four hours of care. I'm so impressed at how researched she is in novel and alternative therapies that may make the slightest difference in the life of someone with a brain injury. In fact, she's more knowledgeable than many pediatricians are on the subject. Despite their caution and their insistence that there's really nothing to be done to improve Benson's outlook, Stephanie is adamant. She's more determined, more educated on his diagnosis than any parent they've ever seen before. She simply refuses to give up when, I think, many parents would have.

Stephanie's dedication to Benson, his growth, and his survival is one of the most inspiring things I've ever witnessed. I know she's always been a fighter. Sometimes I think that by giving Benson those dismal odds, the doctors knew it'd truly motivate my friend. She always says, "They don't know my son." But I know her, and it turns out that toughness has proven to be genetic.

I took my defiance and my fighting spirit with me and built it into my treatment plan when I was diagnosed with cancer. True, I had doctors who shared with me a grim diagnosis and slim chances for survival, but no one doubted me more than my first therapist: the person who was supposed to comfort me the most gave me the fire I needed to defy the odds.

After my original diagnosis, I met with a social worker to discuss the impact of my terminal diagnosis on my mental wellbeing. As expected, I was distraught, confused, and emotional about my new normal. I wanted to gain some perspective about what would lie ahead. I talked to her about my fear of not getting married or having a family. I also told her how important it was for me to finish business school and to finish what I had started. I was only one year into my education, but it had been an enormous goal for me. I wasn't your typical marketing professional or finance guru. I was an older student, a nutritionist with no formal business education, and I really wanted to take my career to the next level. And I had gotten accepted into the school of my dreams.

I shared my concerns with her. I was worried about my treatment schedule conflicting with my schooling. How could I work it all out? She looked at me incredulously. "Are you sure you want to keep going to school?" I was stunned. Why would I stop? This was a journey meant to be finished. I loved school and learning. I had been accepted into a program I loved and was learning alongside a network of students I admired. Was she really asking me to quit?

"I just think you should consider dropping out of school and really think about what's most important right now. I'm not sure how much you realize this, but your illness is very serious."

Each person has the right to make their own decisions about their treatment, and I would never begrudge someone for altering their life's plans upon impact from a traumatic event or illness. But for me, the deviation from my plans, from my personal normal, was as good as giving in to my illness. Having goals, a true north, was something I relished during treatment. Continuing in school was one way I could say, *Fuck off, cancer, I have bigger plans than this.*

From then on, I committed to finishing school on time and with my class. I'd bring my books with me to chemo treatments and share my studies with my nurses. I was supported 100 percent by my classmates and teachers. I even weaved in the cancer business and healthcare industry for several class projects. Sure, I could have waited or delayed, and no one would have faulted me. But *because she told me I couldn't*, I had to. The defiance has helped propel me; it's fueled my inner fire. I truly believe that if someone hadn't told me *no, you can't*, I wouldn't have had the confidence to say *hell yes, I can.*

I went on to finish business school and walked across the stage, on time and with my peers. I'm proud of what I have accomplished. Proving people wrong has become a way for me to exert control over my destiny, and over my illness.

Tell me what I can't do, and I'll show you what I can.

CHAPTER 6

FINDING PURPOSE

I walked up the stairs to the recruitment office just outside of Baltimore with jumbled thoughts in my head. I was leaving the next day to visit friends in Germany and spend three weeks in Europe. I'd put this off for weeks, but it was time to finally commit. My palms were clammy, and I was alone and anything but certain. For some reason, I just kept walking.

In 2010, at the height of the conflict in Afghanistan, I decided to commission into the United States Army Reserve. I'd already been through college, completed my master's degree, and was four years into my career working as a sports and wellness dietitian. But something was missing in my life. I happened upon an online ad in search of part-time dietitians: "*The U.S. Army is looking for Registered Dietitians. Enhance your career and support your country!*"

I had very little exposure to the military. My father was in the Army National Guard for a couple of years, but never saw combat or really anything beyond weekend drills and summer camps at Fort A. P. Hill. Virtually no one in my social circle had served in the military. But something about the ad compelled me. I was twenty-nine and living with my best friend in Northern Virginia. I still don't know why I called that recruiter, but something inside me needed nourishing.

The oath of office ceremony went by in a split second. Within a few minutes, I said those words that committed me for the next eight years to the United States of America. The Captain who swore me in looked me dead in the eye. "I hope your family is ready for you to deploy," she said.

My heart skipped a beat, nerves piling up inside me. At this time, medical units were being mobilized and deployed left and right. Even though I was going to be a nutritionist, my combat experience likely limited, I was still a soldier first. Deployment was a real possibility. After I took my oath of office, I remember going to my car and bursting out into tears. I hadn't told my family I was joining. I hadn't shared the news with almost any of my friends. I'd never been so uncertain about anything in my entire life.

It took a few years, but eventually, I got used to wearing combat boots. I served in two units, a hospital battalion out of Richmond, Virginia where I got to learn under an empathetic and supportive commander, and work with soldiers on their health and fitness. Later, I joined a Combat Support Hospital that was assigned to provide medical and health services to low-income communities across the country. This second assignment was, to this day, one of the most fulfilling parts of my career.

I ended up serving for almost eight years in the Army Reserves. I was part of four rural health training missions where I got to work with people who'd never spoken to a nutritionist before. These people were the salt of the earth, kind, genuine, and undoubtedly hardworking. But they'd never been told saturated fat could exacerbate their heart disease, or they should monitor their carbohydrates because of their diabetes. They had such limited exposure to the most basic principles of health. The time I spent working with them was some of the most rewarding I'd ever experienced, simply because I'd found a way to be useful.

Prior to the Army, I'd worked primarily with people I'd consider privileged: folks who wanted to lose weight, gain muscle mass, or avoid disease. The Army brought me face-to-face with communities who were struggling to survive with the basic tenets of life. I was able to talk to them about how a few changes in their diet could have a profound effect on their lives. I wasn't coaching them on the newest low carbohydrate trend but helping them navigate a $40 monthly food budget while still providing them with adequate Vitamin B12.

I remember one patient I met at one of my missions in upstate New York. She was newly diagnosed with both a food intolerance as well as congestive heart failure. She had no idea where to start, although she knew she needed to change her diet to save her life. Unfortunately, she couldn't afford to work with a health coach. We spent time talking about her diet and her exercise plan. We planned for how she'd eat at home, make meals ahead of time, and use spices to flavor food. Although it was nothing special, I think she appreciated that I was her advocate, someone there for truly her benefit.

A year later, I returned to upstate New York for my annual mission, this time in the neighboring county. A few days in, and my old patient was back. She'd made an appointment with "the dietitian," hoping it was me. She'd changed her entire life, losing over thirty pounds and reducing her cholesterol by almost half. She wasn't there for any reason but to find me and say thank you. She told me that our hour together saved her life. I had to hold back tears. My heart was full. For the first time, I felt like I was doing something that was truly necessary.

The Army sets up these training missions, officially called Innovative Readiness Trainings, across the country, but they rarely receive press. We don't charge for our services. The clinics are set up for a few weeks, and they provide the community with free dental care, medical checkups, vision screenings, custom eyeglasses, and even spaying and neutering of their pets. Since most of the Army Medical Corps is made up of reserve units, organized to be ready for deployment at any time, we're required to have an annual training to keep our skills fresh. Instead of monotonous military drills, units like mine participate in these joint community clinics to ready the troops for wartime, as well as provide a valuable service to communities in need.

When I was diagnosed with cancer, I realized it was time to hang up my boots. I was no longer deployable and, therefore, not a viable component of the United States Army. I had just been selected as a Major but received my medical discharge before I was able to pin on my new rank. Knowing that I didn't *have* to do this anymore was a relief. No more early mornings, no more five o'clock in the morning cadence runs, and no more being told what to do. But I couldn't shake the feeling that I'd lost my purpose.

It's rare to have the feeling of complete connectedness, like your actions are meaningful and making a true difference in the lives of others. Living a life of purpose feels real, alive, clear, and authentic. It's a sense of total absorption that is unlike the mundane of the every day. This sense of purpose helps provide benefits to the soul and mind unlike anything else.

Your life's purpose is the central motivation for your life—the reason you do the things you do, the reason you make the decisions you make. Purpose helps to guide our decisions, influence our behavior, shape our goals, and create meaning in our lives. Often, purpose is connected to our work, which is why we choose occupations that fulfill us. But others find their purpose in other ways, such as volunteer work, spirituality or religion, or even family.[34]

Purpose is unique for each of us, and it can shift throughout our lives. Most important is recognizing that each of us has gifts that are valuable to other people or to our world, and that those gifts are worth sharing.

My friend, Teressa, had to experience profound loss before realizing her need for purpose. I'd known Teressa from graduate school; both of us were working on degrees in nutrition. She and I had a good friendship but lost touch after each of us moved away from Pennsylvania. After college, she embarked on an interesting journey. She became an Eagles cheerleader. She married a former Marine and star UFC fighter. They traveled around the world for his fights and eventually for his sports commentator gigs. They had three gorgeous girls. They were living in a stunning house in Georgia. Their life was, seemingly, perfect.

But at Christmastime in 2011, Teressa recounts a moment that shifted the trajectory of her entire life. She was heading home to Pennsylvania for the holidays. Just before she boarded the plane, her father called to tell her that her brother, Lou, was missing. "I'll never forget getting on that airplane with the level of uncertainty I felt in my heart," she

---

[34] Barb Leonard et al., "Why Is Life Purpose Important?" *Taking Charge of Your Health & Well-Being* (blog), accessed September 1, 2020.

said. He'd been gone for more than twenty-four hours. In her heart, she felt like something was wrong, but she put it off. "I thought, he's probably just at a girls' house. Maybe his phone died," she said. Lou was pretty independent, truly did his own thing. It wasn't unusual for him to disappear when he wanted to. Still, twenty-four hours was a long time, and Teressa couldn't shake the feeling that something was different this time. For two long hours, she agonized on that plane ride, the uncertainty of her brother's fate hanging heavy in the recycled air.

Once they landed, Teressa and her husband headed to baggage claim as quickly as possible, still checking voicemails and texts incessantly. Finally, her husband connected with her father. With his phone up to his ear, he looked over to Teresa, and tears started to form in the corners of his eyes. "I'm sorry, they found your brother, and he's gone."

"The thing is, you just can't process that," she shared. Teressa's brother had taken his own life. Her baby brother, two years younger than her, was gone seemingly out of the blue. Teressa and her family were left with an abundance of questions. None of them felt capable of handling the uncertainty of their feelings or the multitude of frustrations they'd face over the next few months and years. Eventually, Teressa resigned herself to this simple phrase. "You only know what you know." She'd come to accept that there were things she didn't know about her brother, things she couldn't have changed, and things she couldn't have known. Instead of beating herself up about his potential warning signs, she decided she needed to do *something* to make sense of this tragedy.

Teressa's twin sister, Karla, was working at the time as a high school health and physical education teacher. After their brother's death, the two of them started talking about

Lou's struggle with bullying as a teenager. They'd witnessed what they'd consider harmless bullying but realized that Lou may have been harboring feelings of depression for quite some time. The onset most likely occurred around his high school years. While Karla has an opportunity to talk to teens about nutrition, fitness, and wellness during her school curriculum, they rarely talk about mental health. Teens grow up thinking that mental health issues are something that only "crazy" people face or something you shouldn't talk about with others. They began to realize there was a gap for young people and their need for true mental health.

The two of them devised a plan. If they could share their brother's story with young people and increase their exposure to the concepts of mental health and depression, could that improve high school culture on emotional health? Could that reduce the stigma around mental health or decrease the incidence of bullying? Teressa began thinking about the ways that Lou's life could be memorialized in a productive way. So she began to plan. In an instant, her entire life's purpose began to shift. Her motivation was palpable.

In truth, the value of purpose on a person's own wellbeing is limitless. In addition to emotional and psychological benefits, having a strong sense of purpose can actually help improve your health. A 2009 study of over seventy-three thousand Japanese men and women found that those who had a strong connection to a sense of purpose tended to live longer than those who didn't.[35] Additionally, in his study of "Blue Zones," which are communities across the world where people are more likely to live past the age of one hundred,

---

35 Ken Mogi, "This Japanese Secret to a Longer and Happier Life is Gaining Attention from Millions Around the World," *Make It* (blog), *CNBC*, May 22, 2019.

Dan Buettner identified that most of the people who lived past one hundred years old shared a strong sense of purpose. In fact, having a sense of purpose appears to have an effect on all causes of mortality.[36]

In addition, purpose may help to prevent the exacerbation of several specific diseases. A 2008 study showed that lower levels of purpose was associated with earlier death as well as the onset of cardiovascular disease in adult men. More research in this area showed that purpose may have actually been cardioprotective, preventing against heart attack among those with coronary artery disease.[37] In addition, a neuropsychologist at the Rush Alzheimer's Center in Chicago found that those with a low sense of purpose in life were more than 2.4 times more likely to be diagnosed with Alzheimer's disease than those with a strong purpose.[38]

Finally, purpose also seems to even influence our relationships. A 2009 study assessing the purpose of over one thousand adults found that those with a high sense of meaning and purpose in life spent more time on their loved ones, as well as in their communities. In general, people with a strong sense of purpose tended to be more engaged with their families, colleagues, and neighbors and experienced more satisfying relationships as a result.[39]

---

36 "The Minnesota Miracle," *AARP Online* (blog). Accessed September 1, 2020.

37 "What's Your Sense of Purpose? The Answer May Affect Your Health," American Heart Association News, October 8, 2019.

38 Patricia A. Boyle et al., "Effect of a Purpose in Life on Risk of Incident Alzheimer Disease and Mild Cognitive Impairment in Community-Dwelling Older Persons," *Archives of General Psychology* 67, no. 3 (March 2010): 304-310.

39 Neal Krause, "Meaning in Life and Mortality," *Journal of Gerontology Series B: Psychological Sciences and Social Sciences* 64, no. 4 (June 2009): 517-527.

My time in the Army was one of the most purposeful of my life for an abundance of reasons. People are often surprised when they see my resume, or when I share a story from my Officer's Basic Course in the 115°F heat of Texas. Perhaps I'm not, at first glance, a stereotypical soldier. But my time there was incredibly meaningful. The people I met in the Army medical corps were some of the most altruistic, caring people I'd ever meet. Nobody was serving because they wanted money, fame, or recognition. They were serving because it meant something. They were serving because it was their way to make a small difference in the world.

A part of me regrets that I never deployed, which is a crazy thing to say (I know). My area of specialty wasn't particularly useful at wartime, but many of my Army colleagues did serve overseas during wartime. They weren't spending time on the front lines, but they were sewing up casualties in Afghanistan or providing mental health assistance to soldiers in Kuwait. The work they did for our troops was thankless, and they are forever my heroes.

Since my medical discharge, I've struggled to find a purpose as meaningful as the work I did as a soldier. Completing a business degree or getting a job with a Fortune 200 company only helps to satisfy goals, but it doesn't give me the same sense of purpose as serving my country and my community. When I got sick, I knew I had to find a new purpose, something that would also help me feel like I was putting my efforts toward something meaningful. I wanted it to be something that would fulfill me and make me feel like I was doing good for others, something right. In the end, that was the Willow Foundation, and the reason for me writing this book. While it's not the same as my service, knowing I'm doing even something small for others helps fuel my happiness, and in turn, bolsters my own resilience.

Over the next ten years, Teressa and Karla built the Lou Ruspi, Jr. foundation from the ground up. Their mission is to improve mental health and suicide prevention through interactive and educational programs to school districts and communities. Their program is based on several pillars, from spreading optimism, to kindness campaigns, to positive self-care. Thanks to donors, Teressa and her team can provide these seminars and services to school districts on the East coast for free. To date, over fifty-seven thousand students, teachers, and adults have received education and motivation from their team.

Teressa tells me that Lou was a charismatic and outgoing young man. He had a loud, deep laugh and a bright, joyful smile. He loved his family, particularly his sisters, and loved the outdoors. But Lou managed environmental and health issues that escalated over time. Teressa describes it perfectly, "His bucket started filling when he was young. Each issue or altercation was another drop in the bucket. As he got older, because he didn't have the means to face his depression, he wasn't able to drain his bucket," she shared. Lou didn't have one thing happen to him to cause his overwhelming depression, but he wasn't able to manage his mental health in a productive way. His bucket finally overflowed.

The stigma surrounding mental health issues and a lack of publicly available information and education is likely what caused Lou to avoid a proper mental health diagnosis. Teressa believes that Lou didn't want to end his life but that he simply wanted to end the pain. In this way, Teressa knew she had to change her life's focus to ensure others like Lou wouldn't experience the same trauma. If she was able to prevent one suicide from happening, it'd all be worth it.

Teressa's entire world changed the day her brother died. Not just because she lost one of her favorite people in the world but because she eventually found her purpose. Teressa would do anything to bring her brother back. This newfound purpose means that his life and death weren't in vain. The LRJ Foundation has helped thousands of students gain the courage to open up, gain skills, and even get help before it's too late. In that sense, because of Lou, many people out there are finally thriving.

It's a good lesson for all of us. We don't have to tie our personal value to people, to our jobs, or to our achievements, but it's a good idea to find things that bring you purpose. Whether that's an organization you're passionate about, experiences, or causes, finding a purpose helps bring your life meaning. With meaning, you're able to find more peace and satisfaction in your life.

CHAPTER 7

COMMUNITY

The summer after I graduated from college, I started an internship at a weight-loss camp where children were practically forced to lose weight over the course of eight weeks. My internship was one of the most interesting and maddening experiences of my life. But it exposed me to human emotion and connectedness like I'd never experienced in the past.

Movies like *Heavyweights* and TV shows like *MTV's True Life: I'm Going to Fat Camp*, made the moniker "Fat Camp" commonplace in the early 2000s, but I ventured to the summer camp genuinely interested in how a controlled community could truly shift behaviors. I had just received my bachelor's degree in exercise science and was heading to graduate school for nutrition in the fall. Since weight loss was the perfect intersection between nutrition and fitness, I was excited to get a job as a counselor at the camp. I not only lived with and supervised the campers, but I helped with a variety of activities while I was there. I taught basic nutrition classes, helped with the tennis lessons, and taught aerobics. Because of the constant chatter around weight and weight loss strategy, and the constant emotions they'd bring out of the kids, it was an extraordinarily unique experience.

On my first day at the camp, I became acquainted with the surrounding area. Our campsite was in the Pocono Mountains of Pennsylvania on an idyllic piece of property. Lush pine trees were scattered among the more than twenty-five cabins, each one only a few steps away from a pristine, private lake. This camp was clearly primed for elite, wealthy families. For an eight-week stay, the average tuition was close to $10,000.

Before campers arrived, I got to learn the ropes. Since I was going to be teaching nutrition, I'd also help with the weekly weigh-ins, as well as the regulation of the daily food consumption. Each day, the kids would be provided with meals and snacks that totaled about 1,700 calories. They'd eat breakfast, lunch, snack, and then dinner. At night, they'd be allowed to purchase calorie-free beverages, such as Diet Coke or Diet Mountain Dew. In addition, the kids were expected to participate in five different activity periods a day, one of which was always aerobics (for girls) or calisthenics (for boys). Other activities included tennis, golf, a high ropes course, a zip line, swimming, lake activities like jet-skiing, nutrition classes, cooking classes, group therapy, and more.

I was assigned to live with the oldest group of girls; the twelve campers in my cabin were between fifteen and seventeen years old. I quickly realized this was likely the most challenging group in the camp. These young women were dealing with a lot more than just sensitivities about their weight—from wavering emotions, to bullying, to surging hormones. Within the first week, my co-counselor was caught smoking behind the aerobics barn and her employment was immediately terminated. Instead of rehiring another counselor, I was asked to look after the young ladies on my own for the rest of the summer, which was quite an emotional load to bear.

The camp was a hotbed setting for a big group of teenagers, rife with conviction, emotions, and uncertainty. I spent much of my time helping girls deal with their feelings, manage how to talk to boys, and develop an improved body image. Looking back, I cringe when I think about how we'd weigh our campers each week, with the owner of the camp present, and how the camper would receive either encouragement for a successful week of weight loss or a mild lashing for not trying hard enough. I saw the obsession over weight and size blossom in the minds of these young ladies, and how their emotions weighed heavily on what the scale said each week.

I also saw defiance skyrocket as children would order pizzas to be delivered to a stump in the middle of the woods where no one was around, and a black-market snickers bar would go for $10 a pop. These kids, whatever their ages, were managing a roller coaster of feelings tied to their cravings and their weights. The camp itself was emphasizing one simple metric to determine success or failure, which was hard to watch. Yet this was the early 2000s, and we hadn't even started to embrace body positivity as a society. In my naive mind, I simply thought this was an environment where kids could go to get healthy, and it was my job to help them.

Despite my remorse about our tactics, I think back on the experience fondly. The kids were all there willingly, despite the potential pressures they were receiving from their families. They found a certain bond with each other that I'd never seen before. Sure, put kids together in a tight environment for an entire summer and you're bound to see a community form, but the way these kids were able to support each other was uncanny. I was in awe of their strength and determination.

Every kid at the camp was there with one goal: to lose weight. It's a tough goal for anyone, but add in the competitiveness of teens and expectations of parents and you're fit for emotional disaster. I was surprised at how these kids handled the pressure of the camp expectations. The girls I lived with were fast supporters of each other. They identified with their struggles, including how one week they might lose five pounds and the next, gain two. The emotional turmoil over the eight weeks could have torn apart friendships, but I simply saw them bring kids together.

One of my favorite kids, Alison, had a complete transformation during her time at camp. She was one of the heaviest kids that year. She was thrilled when she immediately lost a significant amount of weight at her first weigh-in. The camp was pretty foolproof in that way. Isolate people from certain foods and force them to exercise for several hours a day and you'll always see results. More importantly, I saw Alison blossom socially. She'd come to the camp a total introvert, without friends or much self-esteem. I'd talk with her extensively about her life at home. She didn't grow up rich. Her family had scraped together money to send her to this camp because they were terrified for her health.

She was only fifteen, and she had just been diagnosed with type 2 diabetes. The younger a patient is when diagnosed with type 2 diabetes, the worse their cardiovascular disease prognosis and the shorter their lifespan. In fact, individuals diagnosed with diabetes at age forty or younger have a more than twofold greater risk for total mortality, a nearly threefold higher risk for cardiovascular mortality, and a more than fourfold greater risk for heart failure and coronary heart disease.[40]

---

40 Michael O'Riordan, "Younger Type 2 Diabetes Patients Face Higher Mortality and CVD Risks," *The Heart Beat* (blog), April 10, 2019.

Yes, Alison became an incredible success story over those eight weeks. She lost a ton of weight, gained confidence, and grew into herself while she was at camp. She was able to fit in with the rich, spoiled kids whose parents were off gallivanting in Europe for the summer. She fit in despite the fact that she was the heaviest girl in the camp. Instead, she fit in *because* she was different from them all.

Alison was kind to others. She worked hard and smiled often. She complimented other kids when they were struggling. She told people she loved them. She listened hard. She was thoughtful in her responses. She was optimistic. She was authentic. By all accounts, because of the weight stigma she endured, Alison should have been the least popular camper. Instead, she became the most popular camper.

Alison's positivity didn't come without insecurity. We talked at length about the bullying she'd endured over the years, almost always being the heaviest girl in her class. She'd never had a boyfriend, nor did she think she had a chance to link up with any of the boys at our camp. Nevertheless, she persisted each day with a smile on her face. She didn't come to camp simply to lose weight. She wanted to find a community. For eight weeks, her support and positivity spread like wildfire. If she complimented a girl she didn't know, I could see the immediate impact on her demeanor. If she worked harder in aerobics, other girls around her would too. Her passion spread like wildfire. If she danced with reckless abandon at one of the social events, the other kids would join her, not make fun of her.

She had something about her, something inside that drew others toward her. The support and love she shared outwardly were contagious.

I've thought about Alison over the years and have often wondered how she was doing. Despite the camp giving her a partial scholarship to return the following summer, her family couldn't afford another year of tuition. I lost touch with her over the years, but her attitude and commitment to community have stayed with me.

In thinking about the pillars of resilience I find most powerful, one concept continued to roll through my thoughts: how community is so important in building strength and resilience, and also how hard it is to quantify its value on our overall wellbeing. In researching this book, I turned to my good friend, Shelby Moran, who's a cultural anthropologist and had worked with me on employee engagement and community when I worked at Marriott International. I asked Shelby about our need for community, and why it's poised to be a primary pillar in our ability to rebound from adversity. She pointed me toward our basic human needs, which progresses from physiological needs such as food, water, and safety, to love and belonging, to esteem, and eventually to self-actualization. Shelby believes these needs can each be a ladder to both personal wellbeing and resiliency in the face of adversity. She also believes that the concept of community can help bridge the gap of needs when the individual is deficient. For example, self-esteem and confidence are partially influenced by others. In fact, most of us achieve our esteem from external influences.

While it can be said that esteem should and can come from within, more often than not, our ability to achieve esteem is dependent upon the cultural values of the area in which we grew up or currently live. A global study overseen by Maja Becker found that self-esteem in particular "seems to be mainly collaborative." In fact, her findings suggest that the system for building self-esteem is an important channel through which individuals internalize their culture's values at an implicit level, even if they claim not to subscribe to these values. This means our behaviors, and even our susceptibility to resiliency, can be influenced by our community.[41]

The power of community can be the difference in not just someone's resilience but in their will to live. Twenty years ago, my friend, Haley, was young, in love, and determined. She'd just left the safety of her small-town community, a place where everyone knew her name, and had moved to the big city to start her first real post-college job. She was excited! This new job was with a big company whose headquarters population was, unbelievably, about the same size as her hometown.

Soon after moving, Haley found what she thought was true love. Looking back, she sees her naive self, wearing what she calls "the thickest pair of rose-colored glasses known to humankind." She said, "When I'd decided to spread my wings, I was met with a lot of resistance from those in my community. They were protective of me, but also, they were sad, perhaps even hurt, that I was choosing to leave our community. In fact, some friends even challenged my decision by saying I thought I was better than them. Of course, that wasn't true, and it wasn't my reason for leaving; it was for opportunity."

This put a lot of pressure on Haley. "I felt like I could not fail," she shared. This seemed like a reasonable enough goal for her new job, but in the end, Haley felt like she couldn't fail at *anything in her life at all*. So, very slowly, she began

---

41 "Culture Influences Young People's Self Esteem: Fulfillment of Value Priorities of Other Individuals Important to Youth," *Science Daily* (blog), February 14, 2014.

hiding any speed bumps from those in her original community. Fortunately, and unbeknownst to her at the time, she was building a new community with her coworkers at work. But even they weren't able to predict what would happen to Haley. She found herself in a relationship with someone she thought was the "one," but, "Little did I know," she said, "the 'one' had a completely secret life."

Early one morning, Haley got a phone call that shattered her life. Her new love, the "one," had been involuntarily committed to a mental health facility on suicide watch. Earlier that morning, he had been found by a neighborhood jogger. He'd attempted suicide. The news came out of nowhere, and Haley was in ruins. *Was she in denial about the state of their relationship? How had she not known how depressed he'd been? Was it her fault that he was where he was?* The guilt she felt was overwhelming.

Haley soon learned that "the one" had a hidden drug addiction that had resulted in his financial ruin. "He'd kept this entire other life from me and all those around him." His addiction took him down a hole so dark he thought he'd never get out. He decided his only course of action was to end it all.

Haley was in complete shock. "I was beyond devastated; I was numb. And then I feared my community would find out," Haley shared. *What would they think of him; what would they think of her?* So Haley went into damage control. She worked overtime to try and save her love, his life, his reputation, and their relationship. In truth, Haley was trying to maintain the fairy tale and prove to her family and her original community that she was *still perfect* and that she could make this new life *work and be a success.*

"I actually did pretty well keeping it together for the first week. But then the physical and mental toll was more than I could bear," she recalled. "The funny thing is, I didn't even see myself falling apart. It was members of my new community, my work family, who did." Her real family, who lived more than one hundred miles away, were easier to keep in the dark. But her "work" family saw her. They saw the dark circles, the puffy red eyes that had exhausted all of her tears, and the shaking hands. "It all came to a head when I was driving from the hospital after an early morning visit, headed to my office. This is a drive I'd done so many times already. While speaking to my boss, she sensed my tone had changed and then heard the panic in my voice. I didn't know where I was. I was lost; on the route I knew so well, I had lost all sense of direction and had no idea where I was."

Haley's boss, Angela, stayed on the phone with her as she panicked. Angela skipped her upcoming meetings to help Haley stay calm and helped her navigate her way to the office. When Haley finally got there, Angela had water and snacks at the ready. But most importantly, she made herself completely available to listen. "I don't remember my exact words in that moment," Haley shared, "but I know it came out of me like a waterfall. I do remember that, thanks to her kindness and insistence on listening, when I was done, I could finally breathe. For the first time in weeks, I could breathe."

With Haley's permission, Angela shared the details of Haley's situation with her new coworkers. Immediately, the offers of assistance came from every direction. "They said, 'I'll take this project. I'll check your emails. I'll write that report. Take some of my PTO.' It was simply amazing." While she had cut herself off from her original community, she had been saved by her new community.

In the moments leading up to this rescue, she was on a path that could have cost her job, her sanity, and her wellbeing. Finally, she realized all that was important.

Haley credits this new community with giving her back a sense of safety. By surrounding her in love and support, they provided her the foundation to find her esteem and face her original community.

"I've always told folks that if you ever need something, don't be afraid to ask your community for their help. Many times, people say, 'I don't want to be a burden or put others out.' I would retort by saying, 'If someone you knew needed something and you could help, wouldn't you want them to ask?'" Haley thinks the answer to that question is: absolutely.

That day, Haley was given an alternative perspective, one that she never saw, but was clearly in front of her. Her community saved her. And so she offers some advice: "Don't be afraid to offer. Offer in specifics and not just generalizations. My team, my new community, offered to help me with specific things that needed to be done to pull me out of the pit I was sinking into. Things that, at that point, I couldn't even see I needed."

We need to lean on our community, and we need to let them in.

Shelby Moran also told me that she understands that most people seek out community because there's safety in numbers. "But it goes beyond the buddy system when you're walking at night," she shares. "Having that connection with others often gives us a sense of purpose that we didn't even recognize we needed. There is a strength there." It's human nature to be a part of something bigger than ourselves. It's why we get so wrapped up in our local sports team, or why we glow when we talk about our college alma maters, or why combat soldiers miss their deployments even after returning to the safety of their home.

Haley and Alison's stories are different. Alison built community by being surrounded by others like her, so she was able to form a community out of commonalities. Although the camp wasn't an ideal location for a teen's personal growth, she was able to find a community where she could feel comfortable being herself. Haley, however, found community by receiving support when she was in crisis. She overcomes the stigma of asking for help and the fear of "burdening" others, leading to a net stronger community, with more resilient members.

Community, for many of us, gives us our strength and support in life. With it, we can find our tribe, our common ground. If nothing else, it makes us feel less alone in this giant world.

CHAPTER 8

MAKING A DIFFERENCE

I remember a dark night just a few weeks into my illness. The weight of the diagnosis was hitting me slowly and in waves. One minute, I'd feel hopeful, the next I'd feel as if I'd completely lost my footing, as if the world was crumbling around me. Many nights, I'd stay up late talking to my best friend, Janine, about my life and potential death. I'd talk about how I was supposed to feel or what I was supposed to do. I brainstormed with her about what life would be like without the future I'd planned: without a marriage, without children, without a family to call my own. I cried a lot. I mourned the life I thought I was going to have. I had to come to grips with my new reality even if it meant an entire life swerve.

I don't want to downplay this at all. The things I've had to come to grips with are devastating. I've lost hope for the life I thought I had ahead of me. I had to *give up dreams* that motivated me to the core. At the start of my treatment, I held tightly to the what-ifs. Over time, letting go gave me peace. It's not that I accepted death; it's that I was finally released from the expectations of life. Everyone else, it seemed, had this sense of obligation to what life was supposed to look like. For me, I'd been given the gift of reality. None of us are guaranteed a future. In some ways, I'd been liberated.

I started to get comfortable with this new vantage point: this new utter truth about this non-guaranteed future. I wasn't sure how much time I had, and I realized that I needed to add a sense of purpose to my life. Despite my many passions in my career, my service in the Army, and my love for my friends and family, I needed to dive deeper into my cancer. I needed to find a sense of purpose specific to my illness so that others with the same fate might have a clearer path in the future.

A few months into my treatment, I went to see my oncologist. I'd gone through my first set of scans since my diagnosis, and I was waiting to hear whether the treatment was working. But in my heart, I knew it was. The lump in my breast had grown so big by the time we started treatment, but after only three rounds of chemotherapy, it was noticeably smaller. I was feeling confident.

"Good news, the tumors in your liver have shrunk by almost half," she shared with me. I was ecstatic because it was, indeed, working. I was fairly confident in my therapy; it had a 60 percent initial response rate for patients like me, so I was thrilled to see I'd be a part of the majority. She did a physical exam and noticed the incredible difference in my breast tumor. "It's working everywhere," she exclaimed. "I'm really pleased with this outcome."

The problem is that people with my type of breast cancer can get false hope. While there is often shrinkage at the start of treatment, the cancer never truly goes away. After a while, the tumors almost always become resistant to the drugs and regrow. Then you must move on to a new treatment. But it's been almost four years and I haven't shown signs of regression. I'm in complete remission, with no cancer being seen on any of my scans. I might just be a part of that small minority who gets to live a long time with this disease—I have all the right indicators. I remain hopeful for the future and thankful that the drugs are working.

But I always wonder: why me? What did I do differently? Was my body more primed for the drugs? Or did my lifestyle play into my success? Janine and I have talked at length about this. During chemotherapy, I put myself on a diet that I felt would create the best environment for tumor cell death, but it was based on very, very limited studies. This frustrated me because I felt confident that my diet and lifestyle truly could make a difference in my overall success. But I couldn't find the literature to back it up.

However, I was ecstatic that I was thriving. I started to be more open about my illness with friends and extended family, and the offers to help started to pour in. So many people offered to drive me to chemotherapy or to doctor's appointments, sent me food, made me dinner, or took me to get ice cream. Those I wasn't as close to offered me money. I gathered that they thought contributing something showed that they cared. In a way, they wanted to be a part of my journey. I was overwhelmed with gratitude, but I didn't want the money for myself. My insurance was comprehensive, and I continued to work full time. But I wanted to parlay that generosity into something good, something that helped cancer patients, and something I was passionate about.

So Janine and I founded the Willow Foundation. The Willow Foundation is dedicated to raising money to support researchers focused solely on the complementary therapies that we believe can make a difference in helping people with advanced cancer reach remission. We've funded a handful of researchers who only work at established cancer centers, develop clinical studies, and publish peer-reviewed research that shows the value of diet, exercise, and mindset on the outcomes for advanced cancer patients. While we're still small, we've funded a smattering of researchers across the world who feel as we do: that these studies need to happen. Since drug companies have the ability to patent and monetize their therapies, we know how important it is for these researchers to develop a methodology to improve patient lives, despite their inability to profit from their discoveries.

While I fully believe that we're making a difference with our foundation and I'm excited to see where it goes, I also know that adding this level of purpose to my life helps me to build my own resilience and better enables me to fight my own fight. I was able to find a small way to make a difference in the lives of others, and that's been cathartic. This cause has given me a greater understanding of myself and others and has helped to clarify what really matters.

In general, people report feeling a greater sense of inner peace and satisfaction with life when they're helping others, no matter what it is.[42] Being able to make a difference, despite the size of the contribution, is necessary for human health and wellbeing. Studies suggest that by helping others, you enable a more resilient mindset and have an improved ability to recover from adversity. Helping others stimulates happiness not just to those who benefit, but for you too.[43]

A study by Dr. Thomas A. Plante found that people can cope with stress better when they serve others and connect

---

[42] Sander Van Der Linden, "The Helper's High," *Odewire* (blog), December 2011.

[43] Thomas G. Plante, "Helping Others Offers Surprising Benefits," *Psychology Today* (blog), July 2, 2012.

with others in need. He studied college students attending spring break immersion trips where they worked with those who are poor and marginalized, and assessed their resilience, compassion, stress management, and empathy before they left for the trip, when they returned, and several months later. Those who went on the community service-learning experiences managed stress over time better than those who did not. Dr. Plante believes that this finding is due to a better perspective. "When you have a sense of how much of the world lives, you have a better perspective on life as well as the hassles and challenges of our lives too. Additionally, you experience more empathy, compassion, and solidarity with others as well," he said.[44]

Dallas, also, has been able to parlay his accident into something meaningful. Not long after he returned to Washington, DC after his long stint in rehab, he was quick to prioritize others during his return to normalcy. He knew he wanted to connect with other people who'd had a spinal cord injury, but he wasn't sure if he wanted to do something on his own by starting a new nonprofit or join in on an existing cause. Eventually, he connected with the DC chapter of the United Spinal Association. Dallas didn't waste any time getting involved and contributing his skills. Right away, he joined the board, and, with a background in finance, he was appointed the head of their fundraising committee and given a team of five volunteers. For the past three years, he represented his organization at the United Spinal's Chapter Leadership Meeting and was able to connect with other leaders and advocates across the country.

---

[44] S. L. Brown et al., "Providing Social Support May Be More Beneficial Than Receiving It: Results from a Prospective Study of Mortality," *Psychological Science* 14, no. 4 (2003): 320-327.

Dallas feels like this contribution is important for his growth and resilience. "The more I get involved, the more I want to shake things up!" Dallas even founded the Wheel 2 Win fundraiser in collaboration with Georgetown University, which takes place each year and raises thousands of dollars for the United Spinal Association. Teams of three compete in a wheelchair basketball tournament, equalizing the playing field for the able-bodied and those with disabilities alike. Dallas has an incredible ability to motivate people to get involved. His spirit and resilience are contagious, and you can't help but be inspired.

Throughout Dallas' recovery, he was fortunate to have many visitors and supporters. Some of his staunchest supporters include his college friend, Richard Luck, and his family. The Lucks are a family of givers and show up to everything important—from Dallas' various hospitals to annual charity events. Dallas has had a lot of supporters over the years, but the Lucks have been some of the most dedicated to his growth and progress.

In the early part of 2020, the Luck family asked Dallas to come visit them in Richmond, Virginia as they toured a new healthcare facility, the Sheltering Arms Institute. The institute is a brand-new state-of-the-art physical rehab research hospital that will serve those impacted by a spinal cord injury or disability, traumatic brain injury, stroke, and more. Dallas knew that the Lucks were benefactors of the new hospital, and he was thrilled to take part in the tour.

When he arrived at the facility, the hospital executives rolled out the red carpet. They shared the institute's vision and future aspirations with the crew and gave Dallas a personalized tour of the facility. Even though the hospital is still under construction, Dallas was able to don a hardhat and construction vest to get a sense of the modern and state-of-the-art facility. He rolled through the various centers and gyms in his wheelchair. "I didn't think I could have been more in awe of and taken aback by the advanced rehab facilities. But then, we arrived at the spinal cord injury floor."

Upon entering the center, Dallas and his crew were greeted by another team, a photographer, and a celebratory bottle of champagne. Dallas didn't know he had rolled into the unveiling of the Dallas Disbro Ability Center. "It took me a few seconds until I realized what was happening and saw the picture of me and the signage on the wall. I was in shock, and then I could not hold back the tears."

The Luck family had been so inspired by Dallas' attitude and work for the United Spinal Association that they dedicated an entire physical rehab center to him. "It was a moment I'll never forget," he shared. "I can't wait to see what happens at the Dallas Disbro Ability Center, and I look forward to being a part of it."

Dallas was floored by his new legacy. It motivates him in many ways. "The new theme of the ability center is 'Life Beyond Limits,'" he said, "I've always tried to live life to the fullest. This center just holds me to that promise."

While each of us understands the value of helping others, it's important to note that this, in particular, fuels both resilience and happiness. People who volunteer show an improved ability to manage stress and stave off disease as well as have reduced rates of depression and an increased sense of life satisfaction.[45] In addition, helping others improves us overall. A study conducted in the *Journal of Health and Social*

---

45 Peggy A. Thoits and Lyndi N. Hewitt, "Volunteer Work and Well-Being," *Journal of Health and Societal Behavior* 42, no. 2 (June 2001): 115-131.

Behavior showed that volunteering enhances six aspects of wellbeing: happiness, life satisfaction, self-esteem, sense of control over life, physical health, and depression.

Creating the Willow Foundation has been one of my proudest accomplishments, although it comes with no tangible outcomes: no degree, no money, no awards. I never get to see the patient who may benefit from our research. But I believe in my core that it's valuable. It's allowed me to see past the have-nots that demoralized me after my diagnosis and see the value I may be providing for someone else in need. I'm so lucky to have found something to fill the hole in my soul, which I thought would never be repaired.

I'm also positive that this additional sense of purpose is an important contributor to my health, fueling my resilience. At the end of the day, it's pretty easy to help someone in need, no matter how small the gesture. As an added benefit, you'll benefit from that act too.

PART 3

RESILIENCE TOOLS

CHAPTER 9

NOURISHMENT

I learned how to ski just shy of four years old. I'd like to say I can remember the day I learned, but I'll admit that many of my young, happy memories included days on the mountain. It's had a profound effect on my life.

My mom is a skier. She taught herself to ski in her teens on a small hill in the Upper Peninsula of Michigan. My dad learned in his early twenties, but as a social guy, he loved the concept of traveling and skiing with others. As luck had it, they met on a local ski trip in the DC area and, as they say, the rest was history.

My parents committed to a family ski trip every year, albeit sometimes too small, local mountains on the east coast. It didn't matter to me. It's something I looked forward to every year of my life. Never did I think, however, that my obsession would lead me into a virus hotbed, one that would test my health and nutrition like never before.

There's something extraordinarily magical about the ski experience. Most people love the glaringly obvious—the thrill and rush of soaring at a slightly dangerous pace down steep terrain. The experience itself brings me so much joy.

I love the beauty of the mountains, the calm stillness that exists at the very top, and the seemingly endless views you encounter. I love the difficulty of deep powder, big bumps, and scattered trees. Having the ability to master such obstacles with grace is the ultimate empowerment.

I also love the sociability of the sport. People travel from all over to scale mountains and experience the rush of speed as they make their way down the hill. I've met hundreds of people from around the world in gondolas, on chairlifts, at après ski with a mulled wine in hand, each of us enthralled with the sport that leaves us feeling livelier and more vivacious then we do in our normal, everyday lives. Skiing has always brought out the best in me. It makes me feel alive. For several years, I've been able to recruit a group of friends to go in on a weeklong trip to somewhere mountainous just to ski. It's been one of the things I look forward to the most each year.

In March of 2019, still reveling in our trip to Austria a month prior, my friend Adam and I began planning our trip for the following year. We decided we'd venture to the Sella-Ronda area in Italy, renowned for its long runs through quaint Italian towns and gourmet foods. Soon enough, we had nine friends signed on for a trip that was eleven months away.

However, as our trip was upon us, the world was descending into chaos. We had planned on flying into Venice at the end of February of 2020. Unfortunately, due to the impending global pandemic and crisis and recent news out of Italy, we had to change our plans at the last minute. We decided we'd still fly to Venice but travel north to Cortina, which we thought was out of the hot zone for the coronavirus. We knew there were risks, but we were so excited for this trip.

When we left the United States, the State Department's travel recommendation was a level two: *exercise increased caution*. By the time we landed in Venice, it had increased two levels in twelve hours—level four: *do not travel*.

Regardless of the concern, we tried to make the best of it. We settled on a lovely hotel out of the heart of the city. Only a few people were staying there, so we felt like our risk of contracting the virus was low. We spent a few days skiing and enjoying the gorgeous scenery of the Dolomites. We agreed as a group not to spend time with others in the area and to avoid public spaces. After two days, the ski resort started putting up regulations, including restrictions on the number of people in gondolas and chair lifts. Shit was getting real. We decided it was time to escape north to Austria.

It seemed as though everyone had left Northern Italy to ski and party in Austria. People were everywhere, hundreds on each ski slope and even more at the après ski bars each day. The huge snowstorm was quite the windfall for us skiers, and everyone was in good spirits. Our trip was salvaged.

After four days of skiing, we ventured home. The airports were almost empty; the world had started to recede into itself. Walking through the airport, I had an ominous feeling. *Had we made a mistake staying in Europe? Would we be pariahs coming back into the United States from such a hotbed? Had I put myself at risk as someone living with and in active treatment for cancer?* After all we had been through with our consistent change of plans, the fear and uncertainty of our health, was this trip really worth it? *Did I put my life on the line because of my love of skiing? Or was it worth it to take the risk because, life, for me, truly is short?*

As soon as we landed, Adam looked over at us and said, "I'm not sure I'm feeling very well." I froze. There's no possible way he caught the coronavirus, right? We were so safe, we left Italy, we didn't interact with other skiers, we washed our hands twenty times a day, we used bottles and bottles of hand sanitizer. *Could this really be happening?*

Three days later, Adam sent us a text. Sure enough, he had coronavirus—one of the first cases reported in Washington, DC. After a week, six of the seven of us who had gone on the trip had contracted Covid-19. I was the only one in the group who never exhibited symptoms.

Here's the ironic part—I'm also the only one in our group battling a serious illness. Against all odds, I should have been the one to have contracted this virus, knowing now how prevalent it must have been in Europe. I'd been through chemotherapy, a part of a clinical trial just fourteen months before where my white blood cell counts had been low, but for some reason, I was the only one able to fight off the virus. My body—the one so ravaged with drugs and cancer—had proved to be the strongest.

I've hypothesized about this for a while and have talked to my oncologist extensively. By all accounts, I should have gotten the virus. I was undoubtedly exposed, either along our travel route or from one of my travel buddies. Although we were careful, my friends constantly reminded me of my risk. "Be careful, Leah," they'd say. "The disease is more harmful for those with preexisting conditions." Of course, I knew this, but was it possible that, outside of cancer, I was extraordinarily strong and healthy?

For the three years I'd been in treatment, I'd prioritized my health and wellbeing as much as possible. Once diagnosed, I'd committed myself to optimizing my nutrition, using exercise as medicine, and ensuring I had a positive mindset. These seemed to me like table stakes for a positive outcome. Until now, while having control over these variables helped empower me, I wasn't sure if my dedication to my lifestyle choices had made a difference in my health or if I was just one of the lucky ones who responded well to my treatment plan. After this trip, my confidence grew. Something I had put into place was working. My body was a tough, fighting machine, able to handle not just cancer, but anything life threw at it.

At the end of the trip and after a couple of weeks of quarantine, I realized I had made it to April 2020. I had been living with metastatic breast cancer for three years, which is six months longer than the average patient, and my cancer was undetectable.[46] I'd made it over the hump. Although I can't place my finger on why I was thriving, I had to believe that the choices I was making had a distinctive effect on my overall health and wellbeing. Three years later, over fifty rounds of chemotherapy, nineteen rounds of radiation, two surgeries, four removed lymph nodes, and I was not only healthy, but I was strong. *I was doing something right.* Nutrition had to play a role in my ability to beat the odds.

When I first considered writing a book about resilience, I knew it'd have to include elements of nutrition. I've been a registered dietitian for almost fifteen years and I'm passionate about the power of food as medicine. One of my favorite seminars I've delivered over the years for countless organizations is about Superfoods and the benefit of functional nutrition, or food that has a purpose beyond basic nutrition.

But as I dove deeper into the research, I became discouraged. I'd felt similarly when I started my treatment three

---

46 Dian Corneliussen-James, "Speaking Out on Metastatic Breast Cancer," *Metavivor* (blog), November 7, 2014.

years ago, understanding that good, peer-reviewed research connecting diet to improved cancer outcomes really didn't exist en masse. In addition, I started to delve into conversations with other stage four breast cancer thrivers. I'm a part of several online communities where we share our treatments and celebrate our small (and big) wins. You'd assume that this forum would be filled with alternative treatment therapies and riddled with anecdotes on foods and supplements making a difference. But it's really not. I find myself careful about dispensing advice around food, even though I'm an expert.

The thing is, food and lifestyle have become somewhat weapons of shame. According to many individual studies connecting foods to diseases, including obesity and diabetes, the common perception is that we all should have the willpower to heal ourselves. While I fully agree that we can support our health with good nutrition, there just isn't enough research to make wide, sweeping recommendations around foods.

The fact that there isn't as much substantiated literature on functional foods hasn't stopped Stephanie from using food as medicine in her treatment of Benson. While Benson continues to have challenges, one of the biggest areas of concern is his ability to get quality nutrition. Since he uses a G-tube (a tube that feeds directly into his stomach, bypassing his mouth and throat), Stephanie is unable to sit him up when he eats. He can't take large volumes of food at one time, and he can't be moved very much while eating, so he has to be reclined.

Stephanie and her family are very limited in trying to navigate family meals. It takes over an hour for him to eat. They can't go to a restaurant with him, go on hikes with him, or be anywhere there'll be any sort of movement. Despite these challenges, Stephanie is determined to give him an advantage by providing him with a blenderized diet consisting of real fruits, vegetables, meats, fish, eggs, nuts, grains, and oils. This strategy is quite out of the norm because the vast majority of children who are fed using a G-tube subsist on powdered formulas out of a can or pouch.

Stephanie's determination to ensure Benson receives the valuable components of whole foods has made a substantial difference in his health. He does not get sick as often since starting this strategy. His pallor and subcutaneous fat are healthier. He does not vomit as often, and his mucus load has decreased. His nails and hair grow like crazy. He's the perfect weight and height for his age and is thriving against all odds. Stephanie attributes much of his success to his whole foods and plant-forward diet.

Stephanie's research and education about diet's role in her son's success have been somewhat anecdotal, although more research is coming out each day. "While it's important to rely on evidence-based data when providing recommendations, one thing that is fundamental in advancing science is that there's a big difference between newly emerging clinical data and anecdotal evidence. There is a big shift happening in the tube feeding world, and a lot of that has to do with emerging clinical data," she said. By not just being an advocate for her son but a committed researcher for emerging science, it helps Stephanie provide her son with a nutrition strategy at the forefront of care.

In my case, I purposely choose my foods each day with the hope they're helping to fuel my resilience and combat disease. This empowers me, regardless of the limited literature. To that end, there are a few things I've considered to be key components of a healthy, disease-fighting diet. Regardless of someone's current health, enough research around these principles suggests there are true benefits.

Plant-based diets can heal. The value of plant-based nutrition can't be understated. There's a connection between a diet that's rich in whole grains, fruits, vegetables, and legumes with almost all cases of mortality.[47] We already know that plant-forward eating can help reduce the risk of contracting diabetes, heart disease, and certain cancers. But eating plants can also have an effect on current health. More and more studies are connecting the polyphenols and antioxidants in plants with the mitigation of tumor growth and development.[48] We know that the concept of diet influences the risk for the onset of cancer, particularly breast cancer, but a high-vegetable, high-fiber, and reduced-fat diet can actually reduce the risk of recurrence in survivors.[49]

Water is a huge key to better health. Over the years, we've seen an uptick in water consumption as a replacement for sodas, juices, teas, and coffee. Everyone knows that 60 percent of our body is made up of water. So water is crucial to our overall health and wellbeing, but how specifically can water help us fight disease? A few studies have shown that water has a profound effect on our health, starting with our

---

47 "Vegetables and Fruits," *The Nutrition Source* (blog), The Harvard T. H. Chan School of Public Health, accessed September 12, 2020.

48 Bidisha Paul, Yuanyuan Li, and Trygve O. Tollefsbol, "The Effects of Combinatorial Genistein and Sulforaphane in Breast Tumor Inhibition: Role in Epigenetic Regulation," *International Journal of Molecular Sciences* 19, no. 6 (2018).

49 Manas Kotepui, "Diet and Risk of Breast Cancer," *Contemporary Oncology* 20, no. 1 (2016): 13-19.

brains. In fact, a small amount of fluid loss has been shown to impair both mood and concentration, as well as increase the frequency of headaches.[50] Water also has a profound effect on digestion.

When I worked with patients who were battling chronic constipation, I was floored by how many of them lacked adequate water consumption. Constipation, while seemingly just an annoying manifestation in the bowels, can have a profound effect on health, helping to reduce toxicity and prevent several gastrointestinal cancers.[51] Water has been an important component of my treatment plan. I consume a minimum of seventy ounces a day. Since enacting that somewhat arbitrary rule, I've improved my skin, reduced my eye dryness, improved my bowel health, and have generally felt *better*.

Specific foods could have a role in tumor mitigation. There are a lot of food items out there that may play a role in actually mitigating the proliferation of cancer. We measure the capabilities of our food and its performance in mitigating disease using something called the oxygen radical absorbance capacity. Basically, we're assessing how efficient these molecules are at neutralizing free radicals. Free radicals are oxygen compounds produced in the body from a variety of things, such as UV rays, pesticides, pollution, and so on. While we don't know why some of these oxygen radicals impact our health, we do know there are components in food

---

[50] Barry M. Popkin, Kristen E. D'Anci, and Irwin H. Rosenberg, "Water, Hydration and Health," *Nutrition Review* 68, no. 8 (August 2010): 439-458.

[51] "Gastrointestinal Complications (PDQ): Supportive Care – Health Professional Information (NCI)," Michigan Medicine, University of Michigan, accessed September 12, 2020.

that can render them useless in their attack on healthy cells. We call this free radical neutralization. When we're able to neutralize free radicals, we reduce the risk for cellular damage. Free radicals damage our DNA and RNA, potentially causing an overproduction of proteins that may or may not turn on cellular growth.[52] For those with cancer, free radicals may have played a role in the overdevelopment of cells, leading to tumor growth.

Now, if we have a diet that's high in foods that help to neutralize free radicals, perhaps it can help us prevent tumor growth, along with a whole host of diseases linked to oxygen radicals. While there's a lot of research needed to translate the oxygen radical quenching ability seen in petri dishes to actual human body usage, it's safe to say there's no harm in adding these powerhouses to your diet. Some examples of foods that have high free-radical quenching ability are blueberries, broccoli, oranges, dark chocolate, red wine, spinach, green and black tea, and tomatoes. All of these foods are already great sources of vitamins and minerals and should be a regular part of anyone's healthy diet. However, if you're eating to prevent disease, or mitigate the proliferation of further disease, it's a good idea to keep these on your regular rotation.

Vitamin D is crucial to immune health. When I returned from Europe after our coronavirus adventure, I started to notice some literature being published about the role Vitamin D may play in immune health. In fact, a study of patients in Wuhan, China correlated low Vitamin D levels so closely

---

52 Alugoju Phaniendra, Dinesh Babu Jestadi, and Latha Periyasamy, "Free Radicals: Properties, Sources, Targets, and Their Implication in Various Diseases," *Indian Journal of Clinical Biochemistry* 30, no. 1 (January 2015): 11-26.

to severe symptoms of the disease that I started to do my own digging.[53] We already know Vitamin D is crucial in ensuring we have optimal bone health by helping to facilitate calcium absorption. But the Vitamin D receptor is also expressed on immune cells. Therefore, deficiency in Vitamin D is associated with increased autoimmune disorders as well as increased susceptibility to infection. The results of this correlation are so prolific.

Vitamin D is one of the few individual supplements I'd encourage my clients to take each day. While we make Vitamin D on our skin with our exposure to UV light, even absent of the risk of skin disease from UV, it's challenging to get enough Vitamin D from the sun on a regular basis. In contrast, larger doses of daily Vitamin D supplementation have been shown to help express genes that are important for immune function, response to stress, and DNA repair. In fact, data suggests that any improvement in Vitamin D status will significantly affect the expression of genes that have a wide variety of biologic functions of more than 160 pathways linked to cancer, autoimmune disorders, and cardiovascular disease.[54]

Omega 3's can be protective against a host of ailments. Omega-3 fatty acids have been in the news for almost two decades, and for good reason. Omega-3s play a large role in cell signaling and cellular structure, reducing inflammation

---

53 M. Alipio, "Vitamin D Supplementation Could Possibly Improve Clinical Outcomes of Patients Infected with Coronavirus-2019 (COVID-2019)," *SSRN Electronic Journal*, (2020).

54 Arash Hossein-nezhad, Avrum Spira, and Michael F. Holick, "Influence of Vitamin D Status and Vitamin D3 Supplementation on Genome Wide Expression of White Blood Cells: A Randomized Double-Blind Clinical Trial," *PloS One* 8, no. 3 (March 20, 2013).

in the body, helping to reduce blood pressure, reducing the number of triglycerides in the bloodstream, and even reducing the chance of sudden cardiac death.[55] Omega-3s can also have an effect on our immune health and play a role in fighting disease. Omega-3 fatty acids have been observed to reduce the production of molecules and substances linked to inflammation, such as inflammatory eicosanoids and cytokines.[56] Chronic inflammation leads to all kinds of diseases, from autoimmune syndromes, to heart disease, to cancer. Those eating a Western diet are chronically low in Omega-3 due to a lack of consumption of fatty fish. Unfortunately, you don't find Omega-3 fatty acids in a lot of foods. So if you're not eating fatty fish or flaxseed on a regular basis, here's another case for daily supplementation.

While more and more studies connect diet to the improvement of a variety of ailments, my hope is that organizations continue to fund research, enlist patients in clinical trials, and make more definitive recommendations on how to use food as medicine. There's much more to come in this space, and we desperately need it sooner rather than later.

---

[55] Azin Mohebi-Nejad and Behnood Bikdeli, "Omega-3 Supplements and Cardiovascular Diseases," *Tanaffos Journal of Respiratory Diseases, Thoracic Surgery, Intensive Care, and Tuberculosis* 13, no. 1 (2014) 6-14.

[56] Philip C. Calder, "Omega-3 Polyunsaturated Fatty Acids and Inflammatory Processes: Nutrition or Pharmacology?" *British Journal of Clinical Pharmacology* 75, no. 3 (February 2015): 645-662.

CHAPTER 10

MOVEMENT

Atop Mount Evans in Colorado, I felt more alive than I probably ever had before. I wasn't sure if it was because of the cool, thin mountain air or the seven hours it had taken us to summit the mountain. Regardless, I was invigorated in a whole new way.

When my dad turned sixty, he decided to climb every fourteen-thousand-foot mountain in Colorado, which are dubbed fourteeners. I'm not quite sure why he decided on this path. Perhaps it's because he simply loves mountains or because reaching the summit of something so high in the sky is a rush unlike anything else. For some reason, he was determined to complete all fifty-four mountains in ten years. And I was all for it.

My dad has a lot of friends, many of which are hiking buddies. Very quickly, he was able to assemble a calendar of travel to Colorado, knocking out three or four mountains at a time. He was smart, though; he would never hike alone. Knowing this, I raised my hand to join him. If my dad was going to crush this challenge, I wanted to be a part of it.

In the early fall of 2010, I traveled to Colorado with my mind set on completing two mountains. We stayed in a small, beat-up motel in the town of Georgetown. We'd spent a couple of days acclimatizing to the thinner air, but I was still anxious about the climb. My dad had picked out a doozie for us. We'd be climbing two mountains in one day. The first, Mount Bierstadt, was one of the easiest fourteeners to summit. Most could climb up and get to the summit within four or five hours. However, there was a unique option to hike across a rocky terrain, called the Sawtooth, to get to another fourteener, Mount Evans. There had been several reported deaths on this stretch of the mountain, and the traverse required much of the 1.5-mile stretch to be completed on all fours. My dad was convinced this was *the* challenge for us.

We woke up at three o'clock in the morning to eat and reach the trailhead right at sunrise. The first part of the journey was a breeze. It took us just about four hours to get to the top of my first fourteener. The summit was beautiful: a bright blue sky with dotted, wispy clouds streaking the skyline. I stood atop the ridge peering out over a mass of jagged peaks as far as I could see. The view was breathtaking. We rested for a few minutes, and then my dad nudged me. "Ready for the Sawtooth?"

We journeyed down the small trail and headed over to the rocky trail. I looked back at the gathering of people who remained at the top of Mount Bierstadt. Not one of them was continuing onto the second mountain. They'd all balked at the seemingly obvious risk.

Slowly, carefully, we managed along the narrow route, often scrambling on loose rock with nothing but open air just to the side of our hiking boots. One false step and we could be sliding down the side of the mountain. But this kind of challenge only fueled us more. Eventually, after nearly four hours, we made it to the top of Mount Evans. The view was as bright and spectacular as the summit of Mount Bierstadt, but it was made even better knowing the journey was behind us.

This may be an extreme version, but the exhilaration I feel when I'm exercising, particularly outside, is some of my most empowering emotions. Whether it's a rousing game of tennis, a challenging slope of ski bumps, or the calm meditative sensation from stand-up paddleboarding, exercise provides me with a consistent level of satisfaction and happiness. We all know that exercise, or regular movement, has a profound effect on our health. With regular exercise, we're able to mitigate the effect of a host of ailments from heart disease to obesity to even some kinds of cancer. But exercise can actually be a form of medicine, a tool in your chest to fight an existing illness. It's been an important component of my strategy to live longer, even while having a terminal illness.

Anecdotally, it's easy to see how exercise can help improve our health and wellness. After a run, walk, or bout at the gym, you always somehow feel better. That's likely due to the release of endorphins, or the feeling you may have of accomplishment. But beyond the obvious cardiovascular and mental wellbeing benefits, there's a link between regular exercise and a reduction of risk of overall mortality as a whole. Not only is it good for your heart and keeps your bones strong, but exercise also has an effect on our immunity.

While it's not known exactly how exercise increases immune function during illness, there are several theories. Physical activity may flush bacteria out of the lungs and airways. This could help a person reduce the chances of getting a cold or flu. In addition, exercise causes a change in antibodies and white blood cells. White blood cells are the body's immune system cells that fight disease. These antibodies circulate more rapidly after exercise, so they could detect illnesses earlier than they might have before. In addition, the brief rise in body temperature during and right after exercise may prevent bacteria from growing. This temperature rise may help the body fight infection better. Finally, exercise slows down the release of stress hormones. Some stress increases the chance of illness. Lower stress hormones may protect against illness.[57]

Exercise also can influence cancer outcomes. Dr. Lee Jones of the Memorial Sloan Kettering Cancer Center in New York believes exercise should be prescribed to cancer patients similar to drugs to heighten their success rate. In 2019 and 2020, Dr. Jones was the Willow Foundation's annual beneficiary, initiating valuable studies on advanced cancer patients and their clinical response to exercise. While it's clear that exercise can help reduce the symptoms and side effects of cancer treatment, Dr. Jones is also finding that the act of movement may help change the biological chemistry of a tumor cell or mitigate tumor growth. He found that exposure to exercise following the diagnosis of certain solid tumors may decrease disease progression and reduce cancer-related mortality in many cancers, including advanced breast cancer.[58]

I use it as therapy. I believe it not only makes me feel good physically and emotionally, but it's probably helping me live longer. The ultimate win-win.

---

[57] T. M. Best and C. A. Asplund. *DeLee, Drez, & Miller's Orthopaedic Sports Medicine*, 5th ed. (Philadelphia, PA: Elsevier, 2020), chapter 6.

[58] Alison S. Betof et al. "Modulation of Murine Breast Tumor Vascularity, Hypoxia, and Chemotherapeutic Response by Exercise," *Journal of the National Cancer Institute* 107, 5 (May 2015).

Nancy also credits exercise as a primary source of recovery from her bike accident. After a few weeks had passed since Nancy's accident, her doctors exclaimed they were stunned that she was even alive, let alone able to function at all. They could not understand why she was not completely catatonic. But Nancy knows why. She attributes her recovery in part to her state of fitness upon her accident. Her superior lung functioning and established muscle mass absolutely made her stronger than the average accident victim. Nancy soon realized how important exercise was to her recovery as well.

As soon as she could, Nancy started walking. Once she returned home from her rehabilitation hospital, she made a goal for herself. She'd walk to the end of her driveway. After that, she walked to the end of the street. Eventually, she started running. Within a year, she was running over twenty-five miles a week. Let's put that into perspective. Nancy was given an almost zero chance of recovering at all from her accident. In less than twelve months, she was able to run more than most people can under normal circumstances. Her progress was simply outrageous.

Exercise is medicine for Nancy. She knew that the movement would help build back the muscles that had atrophied during her hospitalization. She also knew the release of endorphins would help her with the emotional turmoil she inevitably faced. She always felt good after a workout, despite how hard or long she was able to go.

Nancy is now back to a grueling routine. She runs four times a week, bikes three times a week, and spends time at the gym. While exercise has always been a part of her life, she realizes now how restorative it's been in her overall recovery.

I include exercise in my everyday activities. But it took me a long time to find the way exercise works for me. After years of heavy lifting and training for softball, or running in the Army, I've learned that I not only need to participate in activities that make my body feel good but also satisfy some other personal need. Yoga gives me headspace and peace along with an increase in my flexibility and help in my recovery from my surgeries. Stand-up paddleboarding allows me to embrace the meditative, repetitive strokes in the water along with the strength from vigorous paddling. Skiing provides me with adrenaline and euphoria but leaves me panting after a grueling run through thick glades. Even a hike with my dog allows me to witness the simple joy and pleasure she gets from being outside, while I clear my head and breathe fresh air.

Everyone knows exercise is a crucial part of health. By including exercise in our daily routines, we're at a lower risk of disease. But exercise is also another tool in our resilience toolbox and is a differentiator for Thrivers. Not only can it prevent disease, but it may play a part in helping to cure existing ailments. In addition, the effect exercise has on our brain functioning and emotional health is substantial. At the core, it's something we can do for ourselves each day that's truly for us alone. If we think about it as a chore, it'll never feel fully satisfying. Instead, we should be grateful for our physical abilities and what they can do for our health and wellbeing.

CHAPTER 11

MINDSET

I've had a nontraditional career path. When I was in high school, my favorite subject was biology. I loved learning about the human body and its capabilities. I particularly liked learning about metabolic processes. I was enthralled by how such tiny organisms worked together to make a body run. Who knew learning about tumor biology would be so personally relevant to me later in life?

I decided I wanted to be a doctor. Unfortunately, my spinal tumor and brain malformation made for a frustrating and disappointing early college experience. I experienced so much pain, loss of sleep, and missed classes that I was doing exceptionally poor in school. I was a freshman at James Madison University in Virginia, and I had a GPA of 2.3. At my school, when you're a sophomore, you need to apply to get accepted into your intended program of study. I needed a good GPA to get into the best programs. I knew I wasn't going to get into pre-med with my GPA. I had to forgo any major that had academic declaration requirements.

Luckily, I rebounded quickly. I was even a starter on my school's division one softball team. The team was newly formed due to the college's adherence to Title Nine, which ensured the proper distribution of athletic opportunities for both men and women. I had been recruited to play softball for a handful of schools, but the opportunity to be a founding member of a new division-one team was exciting. My life in college consisted of softball and social events, and that's about it.

Even though I wasn't particularly passionate about my classes, my zest for learning about the human body remained. Eventually, I found a home in the exercise science department. I loved the human physiology classes, the anatomy cadaver lab, and the biomechanics class. But I mostly enjoyed nutrition. Learning about nutrients and how they propel the human body or how compounds found in nature could prevent or even cure disease was inspiring to me. Even better, I loved learning how food affected athletic performance and how the tiniest change in nutrition strategy could boost an athlete's performance, give them more power, or get them past the finish line. I finished my degree in exercise science and went on to receive a master's degree in sports nutrition and exercise science with the intent of working with elite athletes on their sports nutrition strategy.

I didn't realize I wasn't cut out for patient work. The monotony of the interactions grew boring over time, and I felt frustrated that I could only give my patients motivation and education, much of which they were starting to find online. After two years of private practice and four years as a base dietitian at Bolling Air Force Base, I got a job as a corporate wellness consultant at a national firm in the DC area. I was pumped. My job was to work with companies, large and small, to help them develop a strategy to improve the health of their employees. For the next several years, I helped to grow the company, often participating in new product development, but I mostly thrived in client services. I loved what I did, and I loved my coworkers. In fact, there were many days when I worked all night long just to get a project right. I felt immense satisfaction when a client was happy or when our CEO gave me praise, so much so that I craved it.

My boss, Karen, and I never really got close to one another. I respected her, but we had different working styles. She operated without emotion, always putting clients first, and I liked to bring my authentic self to work. We'd try to connect socially, but it somehow felt awkward. Regardless, I liked my job so much I was generally able to ignore any issues that would arise. However, about a year before my diagnosis, we started to have an increase in disagreements.

Each time we'd have a conversation, it seemed like there was conflict. She disagreed with me on the way I managed my direct reports. She preferred more passive-aggressive emails to direct confrontation, which often led to misunderstandings. And I'm sure I frustrated her too. I was a straight shooter, yearning for real talk. She was a pleasant, polite person who didn't ever want to deal with bad news. It seemed like we were destined to disagree.

Looking back, I see the amount of stress I started to develop over the years at that job, but I had internalized so much of it solely due to my poor relationship with one person. I had let my anger get the best of me. Each email Karen sent made my skin crawl. I wanted so much to validate my frustration that I started *looking* for things to prove that she was demeaning me. I was, in a way, trying to be unhappy, and my inability to handle it productively was leaching into my wellbeing.

Two months before my diagnosis, Karen moved me into a new position. I found out later it was because she was frustrated with our challenging relationship, and she needed me to fall under a new leadership structure so I would no longer report to her. With the change in position, I was placed into a sales role with a commission structure, something I was not prepared for, nor desired. I also lost my team and my role in creating productive solutions for companies. I was even asked to leave my consulting relationship with my longstanding favorite client, a local Fortune 200 company.

But as I was training for my new role, I was hit with a diagnosis: terminal cancer. When I shared my news with my new boss, and then with our CEO, they were floored. Luckily, they accommodated me by providing me a new role. I could work on projects and I didn't need to travel or come into the office. I was able to work from home or the hospital during chemotherapy and not lose out on the money I needed to sustain my life. While the company wasn't particularly supportive or encouraging, they more or less left me alone, which I appreciated.

Once I finished with chemotherapy, I entered a clinical trial to determine the effectiveness of a new drug. This drug, coupled with my continued infusions, put me at a total of six cancer medications, two of which I received via port IV every three weeks. Moving from chemo to the trial didn't change much. My hair started to grow back, but the scans still showed cancer. I was still immunocompromised. I still felt unwell and was still fighting for my life.

Two months into the trial, my CEO asked to speak with me. She told me that while they'd been pleased to accommodate me during chemotherapy, it was time for me to move back to the sales position. I was taken aback. I knew that a sales role with frequent meetings and travel wasn't going to work with my treatment schedule. So I resigned. A part of me wonders if that was part of their plan, but it didn't matter. I needed this motivation to find employment where I could thrive. I ended up joining the team with my favorite client.

For the next several years, I found a home at my new company. My team supported me as I continued my treatment. They allowed me to work from home or the hospital as often as I'd like and created a new role that fit my expertise perfectly. Sure, I was just an employee, but it was clear they truly cared about me as a person.

I think about my old job every once in a while. I think about the immense stress and pressure I was under and the time I spent managing my feelings about my position and my relationship with Karen. I can't blame her for everything that went wrong with me there. However, I sometimes wonder if my stress and emotional responses were setting me up for something catastrophic. Three months before my diagnosis, I had visited my doctor and received a breast exam and there was no trace of a lump. My cancer had either grown exponentially or was exacerbated significantly during those three months. Within those three months, I had harbored a significant amount of stress.

Virtually all jobs provide some amounts of stress. For some reason, the stress I accumulated during that time brought me to my breaking point. I truly believe my inability to manage my emotions brought out the worst in me, and I manifested my frustration and anger as an exacerbation of my illness.

Over the past several years, there's been an increasing interest in the correlation between stress and our physical health. While everyone feels stressed from time to time, a body of evidence is mounting that suggests our inability to manage stress may be the cause of or fuel for a variety of ailments.

Stress is how our bodies and brains respond to any demand. Whether someone is facing a challenge at work, a traumatic event, or simple life events such as traffic, our bodies exhibit a physical reaction to these emotional events. However, not all stress is bad. In fact, many of us thrive on stress. Think about your daily to-do list. That list is a challenge you're providing to yourself, something that helps center you and keep you motivated. It may cause stress, but your ability to handle it and knock out tasks helps you build confidence and resilience.[59]

The stress that overloads us is not necessarily different from our positive stress, but it's the physical manifestation of *unhandled* stress.[60] If we're overloaded with challenges, or if we become emotionally drained, the stress of a new challenge can cause a physical toll on our bodies. Chronic stress, or stress that we experience over and over, is particularly dangerous. According to the National Institutes of Health, long-term stress causes the body to never be able to return to normal functioning. With chronic stress, the consistent signaling of the brain that there's something to do, or something to escape, can cause disturbances in the immune system, digestive tract, our sleep patterns, and even our reproductive systems. Over time, this strain on our bodies can contribute to a variety of serious health issues, such as heart disease, high blood pressure, diabetes, and, of course, depression and anxiety.[61]

Teressa knows how mindset can truly impact someone's life. After her brother's death, Teressa dedicated her life to

---

59 "Stress," Cleveland Clinic, accessed September 8, 2020.

60 "Stress Symptoms," WebMD, accessed September 8, 2020.

61 "5 Things You Should Know About Stress," National Institutes of Health, accessed September 8, 2020.

mental health and wellness. Her passion for leadership and empowerment has helped thousands of kids understand anxiety and depression and destigmatize mental health. She understands fully the meaning of a positive mindset and how you can coach yourself to make real improvements.

Teressa spends time thinking about how her brother Lou's life spiraled out of control. She realized he had experienced years of stress and pain that he hadn't acknowledged or managed. That stress ended up overflowing. Even though Lou was an extreme case, Teressa believes anyone, despite their background or exposure to trauma, can harbor pain and anxiety that can lead to serious consequences. While serious matters certainly require prompt attention from mental health professionals, those of us managing daily stressors can add mindset exercises to our daily routine to improve our resilience.[62]

The most important aspect of stress, Teressa shares, isn't the stressor, it's our reaction to it. Emotions are natural occurrences within our body, simply a response to our environment or situation we've encountered. "You could go through a range of emotions throughout the day, from pure joy to rage to sadness. It's simply the way our bodies work," she shared. "We need to understand how we can handle these emotions and not simply push them back down."

"We can handle emotions by talking about them, for starters," she shares. Be open and honest with someone you trust. Your emotions are real and need to be acknowledged. Then work on letting your emotion go. "It's easy to get lost in worry from something that's happened or something that could happen in the future. We take what's happening now for

---

[62] Karen Doll, "23 Resilience Boosting Tools and Exercises," *Positive Psychology* (blog). January 9, 2020.

granted." In other words, try to focus on the here and now, and not the past or future.

This centering helps mitigate emotions or reactions in favor of the big picture. Instead of ruminating, notice what's happening right now. If humans were more apt to search out and notice the small joys in life, from the softness of your sheets at night to the warmth of your coffee, we'd be filling up our resilience cup with positivity. Then we'd be much more poised to handle conflict or adversity later.

In addition, Teressa teaches her students about coping skills. One of the most important things she shares is the importance of *letting go* to help calm nerves and refocus our mindset. "You must be able to walk away from drama," she shares. It may feel hard to walk away from a stressful situation, but it's a muscle we need to exercise repeatedly. Letting go of an altercation, a run-in with someone in traffic, or the stress of a bad grade each time will help build your emotional strength. While it may feel hard to let go when feeling frustrated, the ability to release emotion is one of the most important components of resilience. Each time you're able to walk away, or let it go, you're building that mindset muscle.

Changing mindset is incredibly challenging. But I've implemented a few things that have helped me shift my mindset ever so slightly. I'm more able to see the good in things. I'm more capable of letting the bad go. And I'm more understanding and empathetic as a friend and coworker. Here are some ways you can operate with a mindset of a Thriver:

1. Don't hold grudges. Ruminating on negative feelings or interactions will only diminish your wellbeing and will do nothing for the other person. Whatever issues you have, let them go.

2. Lift other people up. Do things for your family, your friends, and your network. Celebrate their successes as much as your own.
3. Don't make excuses. Take ownership of failures, no matter the consequences.
4. Get absorbed into the present. By being immersed in whatever you're doing, you're giving your mind permission to breathe. Some do this by meditating regularly, but I like to take mini breath-breaks throughout the day. If that's not your style, try adding something creative to your daily routine, like art, lettering, or even puzzles. Add something that doesn't include distractions containing a screen.
5. Look for the good. Find the silver lining. See the bigger picture. Life is too short to be angry.

It's been years since I changed companies, and I've certainly had my fair share of stressors. My jobs since then haven't been stress-free. But I've figured out how to manage my boundaries. I'm far more at peace. I don't say yes to every project. I don't work all hours of the day. If I feel connected to an idea, I'll fight for it, but not at the expense of my wellbeing. I work from home often and sometimes even take short naps in the middle of the day.

I don't have to be the best employee in the company, but I am okay with being a good employee. I love what I do, but it's not all that brings me true joy and meaning. While the world continues to digitize and we see the blurring of life and work, I make it a priority to step away often and focus only on myself and my family each and every day.

CHAPTER 12

LOVE

It's hard for me to talk about this topic, despite how important I know it is. The truth is, I'm both incredibly unlucky and incredibly lucky in love.

First, my unfortunate history. In the several decades that I've been dating, I've never found "the one," or even anyone close. I've had a few relationships, some were positive, and I look back fondly on them. But I mostly had disappointments, men I've dated along the way who have broken my heart before I'd even shared it was theirs to break.

There have been times where I've considered giving up. When I first got sick with cancer, one of my hardest realizations was that, without the certainty of the future, it'd be unlikely that I'd have the chance to fall in love again. I also realized that, due to my medications, I'd never be able to carry a child. In one fell swoop, I mourned the entirety of my future.

Despite this, I've remained eternally optimistic that love will come my way. My friends share this optimism with me: the person who will love me despite my illness will love me because of it. Because I've been able to live with this illness and because I've, hopefully, embraced my life so authentically, the right person will be here in due time.

That may happen and it may not. I've come to terms with that. I've decided to spread and share love so broadly that it'll shine *out of me* instead.

The lucky part of my love life has been my relationship with my best friend, Janine. She's the absolute love of my life.

I met Janine when we were both young and silly, and we were still in college at JMU. We played softball together and, thus, were destined to be friends. How close, I never knew.

Janine is a tough nut to crack. Unlike me, she's an introvert to the core. She hates in-authenticity. She feels like the life is sucked out of her if there are too many people in her presence. She hates talking about herself. She'd rather hang out with the dog at the party than the people. She only has a few close friends. She's warm and kind to everyone but trusts only a select few.

One day at practice, while we were setting up our equipment, we happened upon a little figurine that a child had left in the wire fence. Upon closer inspection, I realized the figurine was a tiny unicorn My Little Pony. Excited, I showed my teammates. "I love unicorns! They remind me of my childhood!" Truly, I had loved the mythical creatures as a young girl, romanticizing their strength and beauty. On a whim as an impulsive, eighteen-year-old on spring break in Florida, I had even spontaneously indulged in a small unicorn tattoo on my right torso.

As I was laughing with a teammate about this cute, strange anomaly of a unicorn, Janine tapped me on the shoulder. I looked at her as she pulled up her shirt just slightly and showed me a tattoo of her unicorn right on her hip. I squealed with delight and showed her mine. We divulged into laughter. I'd found my person.

Janine and I have been friends for twenty years. She, too, has been unlucky in love, and, thus, we've been able to be at each other's beck and call for decades. When I first got the call that I'd been diagnosed with invasive breast cancer, she was there in the room with me. When I found out it had metastasized to my liver, she was there in the car with me. In fact, when I knew that I needed help during chemo and didn't want to move home to live with my parents, she moved out of her apartment and into my spare bedroom. She stayed with me for nine months while I went through my hardest chemo and the start of my clinical trial. Even when she did move out eventually, her condo was only a mile and a half away from mine. She's made it a priority to come with me to almost every single chemotherapy appointment I've ever had, over sixty-five of them, simply to be there with me.

I know that a friend can't substitute for the emotion you experience with a lover and with family, but I am so incredibly lucky to have Janine. Without her, I'd never had experienced the unconditional love each person has a right to experience. Without her, I'd never have the confidence to battle each milestone. Without her, I'd have felt alone. Not because I didn't have friends and family who would have dropped anything to help me, but because she was the only one who actually *wanted to be there*.

Love, in any form, improves our resilience in the face of an emotional or physical crisis. In general, the better-quality support a person can draw on from friends and family, the more flexible you can be in a stressful situation. There's the clear benefit: loved ones in your life will care for you if adversity befalls you. Having a support system will help you have a greater sense of confidence and will allow you to approach life more optimistically.

In addition, the ability to maintain enduring friendships and love appears to be more important for maintaining physical and emotional health in addition to resiliency. Studies have shown that middle-aged people who have at least one friend they can turn to when they are upset have better overall health than people without such a friend.[63] Similarly, single people are at a greater risk for depression than married people, and people who withdraw from social contact when they become ill tend to become sicker. Seen in this light, having a supportive group of friends and family is a major asset for maintaining good physical health.[64]

When I talked to Nancy, I could see that love played a huge role in her recovery from her accident.

Obviously, Nancy had experienced a physical toll unlike anyone could imagine. But the depression she experienced was the most unexpected, frustrating part of her recovery. At one point, Nancy thought to herself, "Why didn't I just die?"

Before Nancy had her accident, she considered herself to be an incredibly positive person. She had a good job, a loving marriage, two great kids, and was a world-class athlete. In one moment, that entire dream shattered in front of her.

As she laid there in her rehabilitation hospital, unable to walk and with sheer frustration, she realized something she'd known all along. The love of her family would be what helped her get through this. "I owe it to my family to try as hard as I can to get better."

---

[63] "Depression and Older Adults," National Institute on Aging, accessed September 8, 2020.

[64] Harry Mills and Mark Dombeck, "Resilience: Relationships," *Helen Farabee Centers* (blog), accessed September 9, 2020.

So Nancy worked her hardest to get back the strength and mental agility she once had. Her husband, Richard, was by her side. He drove her to every appointment, sat with her when she was confused, and coordinated her care. He was her rock.

Her daughter, Elena, was right there too. Elena, a medical researcher, had every clinical study at her fingertips and learned all she could about traumatic brain injuries. If there was a supplement to try or a therapeutic that could work, Elena guided the way.

Nancy's son, my friend Adam, was also there. As soon as they got word that Nancy had been in an accident, he immediately dropped everything and rushed to her side. She was, in one instant, surrounded by love.

Nancy believes the one positive that has come out of her injury is the deepening of her relationships. Before her injury, Nancy thought what every mother has thought: "I love my kids, and they'll always be here for me." But when they showed up and spent months at her side, she was floored. "I got how much they loved me, but I didn't really *get it*. The love they gave me was instrumental in my healing. When I was recovering, I needed support. They became my *team*."

A few months later, Elena gave Nancy another gift. Despite years of proclaiming she never wanted to have children, she and her husband decided to have a baby. Seeing her mom in the hospital, witnessing how fragile life can truly be, she realized she wanted exactly what her mom was experiencing, the true love of a family unit. She decided that she wanted her support too. Just ten months after Nancy's accident, Elena had a baby girl. "It was her gift to me. I got to be a grandmother, and she got to have *her* team."

It turns out that love in any form—whether between a couple or between friends, and even pets—can be an incredibly transformative and fulfilling experience. In addition, love can vastly improve your health in four specific ways.

Love reduces stress. Everyone knows how cathartic it is to get a hug from a loved one after a stressful day or to embrace a loved one when celebrating good news. This emotion, specifically through hugs, can actually lower blood pressure as well as raise oxytocin levels in the blood. Oxytocin levels can increase even when you cuddle with a pet. When these levels are increased, people generally tend to feel more connected and develop bonds with their loved ones. In one study, married couples who held hands significantly reduced stress from anticipated electric shocks when compared to holding hands with a stranger or with no one at all.[65] Even verbal affections, such as saying "I love you," is connected with reduced levels of the stress hormone, cortisol.[66]

In fact, love can help us become more resilient to diseases, as it may improve our immune systems. Love increases levels of Immunoglobulin A, an antibody found in mucus membranes that helps to fight antigens in the body. In one trial, adults who had sex one to two times a week had significantly higher salivary glands of Immunoglobulin A than those who reported less intimacy.[67] The good news for those who are less sexually active is that simply spending time with your pet can also improve your immune function. One study showed

---

[65] "Holding Spouse's Hand May Reduce Stress," *CBS News* (blog), December 20, 2006.

[66] Nicol Natale, "Falling in Love Changes Your Body and Brain – Here's How," *Business Insider* (blog), July 12, 2018.

[67] Carl J. Charnetski and Francis X. Brennan, "Sexual Frequency and Salivary Immunoglobulin A (IgA)," *Psychological Reports* 94, no. 3 (1994): 839-844.

that spending just eighteen minutes petting a dog showed significant improvements in Immunoglobulin A.[68]

Love can also provide relief from pain. In one study of college students in the first nine months of a romantic relationship, looking at a photo of their boyfriend or girlfriend significantly reduced self-reported pain in comparison to looking at a photo of an acquaintance.[69]

Finally, love extends your life. Many studies have shown that having a loving network contributes to both the quality and quantity of your life. In a meta-analysis of 148 studies, those with the strongest relationships had 50 percent increased longevity rates than those with weaker bonds.[70]

I've managed to see past society's obsession with romance despite still yearning for it if it is the right person and the right time. I'm constantly thankful for the love I receive from Janine, my friendships, my family, and even my dog. I think of these life-giving relationships as gifts I've been given that allow me to thrive, and help me feel valued, cared for, and important.

No matter the origin, it's clear that love helps us grow emotionally, helps improve our health, and helps us feel more resilient. Every ounce of love you share with others powers their long-term health and happiness too. It's not a zero-sum game. Be open with your love and give it widely and freely. Your health depends on it.

---

[68] Carl J. Charnetski, Sandra Riggers, and Francis X. Brennan, "Effect of Petting a Dog on Immune System Function," *Psychological Reports* 95, no. 3 (2004): 1087-1091.

[69] Tara Parker-Pope, "Love and Pain Relief," *Wellblogs* (blog), *The New York Times*, October 13, 2010.

[70] Julianne Holt-Lunstad, Timothy B. Smith, and J. Bradley Layton, "Social Relationships and Mortality Risk: A Meta-Analytic Review," *PloS Medicine*, July 27, 2010.

CHAPTER 13

KINDNESS

One of the most meaningful emails I received after I was diagnosed with stage four breast cancer was from my childhood bully.

It's interesting to use that word. I'm not sure that's the term I would have used growing up, or if it even makes sense for what occurred. Bullies, to me, were just mean girls, girls your mom would tell you to ignore. I'd known this girl since the first grade, when she and I were both new kids in our elementary school. Most of the kids in my school started there in kindergarten. However, Erin and I were both new kids together. She was a kind, inclusive girl. I took an instant liking to her.

Over the years, Erin and I waxed and waned as friends, as young girls do. By the time we hit fourth grade, Erin seemed to have made closer friends with a handful of other girls who didn't seem to like me. These girls created a new group of friends, a true clique with their own rules and regulations. I'd ask to join the group, but there was one excuse after another. "You're too tall," they'd say. "Your name doesn't start with E," they'd quip. It seemed the more they wanted to keep me out, the more I wanted in.

Much later, I determined I had a huge need for social connectedness and a special desire for inclusivity. Over the years, my happiness often correlated with whether I had a group of friends to spend time with, enjoy laughs with, or to rely on. The insecurity I felt in my grade school years stayed with me for quite some time, even throughout middle and high school. I always needed a place to belong.

Later in elementary school, I struggled to find a group of friends who I could feel comfortable and confident being around. I found myself yearning to connect with Erin and her crew. A few weeks into sixth grade, Erin started acting funny. She'd coordinate after-school hangouts and sleepovers and wouldn't invite me. She'd whisper to others when I was around and laugh ominously. At lunchtime, there'd never be enough seats for me to join the crew. Finally, she surprised me with a present one day—a mixtape of songs she'd put together just for me.

I was ecstatic. What a kind gesture! I knew Erin still cared about me; she probably was just going through a weird time. Besides, we'd been friends—mostly—since first grade. I took the songs home and started playing them in my boom box. *Cold as Ice* by Foreigner boomed through the speakers. *This is a weird choice*, I thought. *Fat Bottom Girls* was next, followed by *You're So Vain*. On and on the list went, mean song after mean song. I finally got it. Erin was sending me a message.

The interesting thing about twelve-year-old girls is their inability to communicate feelings directly to each other. I'm not quite sure this shifts too much as we get older, but the young, emotion-filled tween brain can't seem to rationally handle conflict and pleasant exchanges with differing opinions. Erin had decided that the best way for me to stop hanging around was by passive-aggressively telling me to *fuck off* via a poorly constructed mixtape. In fact, when I approached her about the tape, she gaslit me incessantly, insisting she just liked the songs and they weren't meant to be mean. Despite us attending two more schools together and eventually playing on the same tennis team in high school, our friendship never recovered. The uncertainty and insecurity I felt about trust and friends stayed with me for years.

Fast forward more than two decades and I find myself at my lowest of lows upon receiving my diagnosis. News of my illness spread quickly among my high school classmates. Before I made any public announcement about my illness and impending treatment plan, I started to receive emails and messages from people I hadn't talked to—or thought of—in many years. Most of the emails were short, kind messages of hope. Some people offered to take me to treatments or send me a meal or care package. Unsurprisingly, dire circumstances often brought out the best of my network and I received a ton of support and love.

And then I received an email from Erin. She had gotten my email address from a mutual friend who had shared it with her without my knowledge. In an instant, I was frozen. What could this person possibly have to say to me at my most vulnerable moment?

In all the years I had known Erin, I had operated with extreme emotional volatility. Little jabs, gossip, event exclusions, passive-aggressive comments—all of these could send me into a tizzy of emotions. I thought of the times that I had yearned for inclusivity in Erin's group: the pain and frustration it brought me, or the times my parents told me to *stop being so sensitive*. They were right to be tough on me. I hadn't built any resilience to emotional turmoil. Each tiny action by a mean girl sent my head, and my emotions, for a tailspin.

Over the years, I had built up my resilience significantly but was still traumatized by the emotions that had been seared into my memory from so long ago.

The email was entitled, "Fight and Light." Erin admitted to me that she had been thinking about me and had a tough time composing her email. She mentioned that our paths hadn't crossed in nearly two decades and that she was probably one of the last people I'd want to hear from. But then she said the things that made me feel the proudest I'd felt in quite some time. "I'm blown away by your bravery and emboldened by your resilience." Was this email written to me? The same person who cried when I lost a tennis match or wasn't invited to a birthday party?

The vulnerability she embraced to reach out to me was all I needed to start to shift my perception of her, to give her the benefit of the doubt. I saw her for what she had become, a kind, thoughtful, and caring woman. I recognized that she had grown, that I had grown, and realized that we could repair what I thought had been lost. I could have been angry about receiving this email. I could have told her that I had plenty of support from people who had been there for me over the past fifteen years. But I didn't. Something inside me melted, and the anger I'd harbored for years began to drip away. My cancer, my crisis, had brought us together. If she hadn't taken the first step, I never would have been able to address the bitterness that had been living inside me.

Erin and I exchanged a few emails over the months I continued with treatment. We even connected at our high school reunion a few months later. We've talked about our interactions as young women and have traded memories and apologies. We talked about the mixtape, and she shared her feelings of guilt and disgust about the entire exchange, her desire to fit in with a new cool crowd getting the best of her. I, too, had treated her poorly at varying parts of my life. Most notably when I chided her for missing a pop fly at our little league all-star game and in high school when I had scored a new group of friends. She remembers me as distant and, perhaps, even dismissive.

Despite the individual accounts of our childhood, Erin has since become a source of support and loving conversation, becoming a cathartic addition to my healing process. Erin was once someone with which I equated insecurity, frustration, and belittlement. But Erin was just a young girl then too. I wondered if there were others in my past who thought similarly about *my* actions toward *them*. As girls and teens, how able are we to be empathetic toward others, to truly understand their feelings and predict their emotions when our own insecurity plays so loudly in our heads?

I've thought about my ability to evolve so significantly over the years. How I've been able to handle the emotional turmoil that my life has brought me when I spent my childhood crying so hard and feeling so deeply. And I think it's not that I haven't lost my sensitivity but that I've been able to use it for good instead.

Yes, things still bother me. Actions of exclusionary friends and hurtful comments can be tough to handle. But these micro-problems help me stay in the present. I'm able to focus on problems in the here and now and determine whether I have the control to make it better. And if I don't, I can let it go. If it's in the past, I can put it behind me. If it's in the future, I can relinquish worry. It keeps my mind on ever-present things, those conflicts and frustrations that make life what it is. Without those downs, how clearly could we appreciate the ups?

I relish in the memories of my childhood and choose to remember the good parts of my relationship with Erin. I remember finding a spot in the woods near her house where we'd steal away from her parents to chat and write poetry together. I remember sleepovers and birthday parties and celebrating our high school tennis team's trip to the state tournament. Most importantly, I remember the courage it took her to write me out of the blue after eighteen years to tell me she was proud of me, she looked up to me, and she loved me.

There's intense power in kindness. For some reason, being kind wasn't the most popular thing to do when I was growing up. It wasn't ingrained in us that we should be kind to the kid who was left out of the sleepover or that we should be empathetic to the child with failing grades. For some reason, we were taught to compete and excel. Our parents left out the part where we needed to lift others up to be truly happy.

Despite the obvious, kindness helps others and repeated kindness can make you a better person. Over time, many of us have gained unkind qualities, from biases to our own insecurities. But the good news is that kindness is a muscle, and the exercises are similar to learning a new hobby. We can actually train ourselves to be more compassionate to others in the face of suffering.

In fact, researchers at the University of Wisconsin, Madison completed a study in 2018 that affiliated compassion training with improved responses to other people, particularly those who were suffering. One group practiced loving-kindness meditation, which is a simple meditation that involves directing well wishes and compassion toward other people, as well as to ourselves. The other didn't. The loving-kindness practice begins with each person working inward on themselves. Eventually, it moves to loved ones and then toward people you don't know. The practice builds a muscle in kindness and compassion.[71]

After two weeks of loving-kindness meditation, participants received brain scans. In the scanner, the participants were shown images of people suffering and also of neutral images. Those who practiced loving-kindness meditation tended to look more directly at the images with suffering and also showed less activity in the areas of the brain associated with emotional distress. These results suggest that compassion training could help people be more compassionate and feel calmer in the face of suffering.

Teressa understands the importance of kindness. In fact, she credits bullying to the stress and anxiety that manifested in her brother. His inability to deal with his stressors led to a deep depression and, ultimately, to taking his own life.

And now, Teressa talks to kids all over the country, not just about the importance of mental health, and how crucial it is to share thoughts and feelings, but also how to be a good friend. Teressa said that children at a young age need to be taught that kindness is cool and being compassionate to others is the right thing to do.

One of my favorite examples she used is a game Teressa plays with her kids. After she's talked to them about kindness and bullying, she tells them they're ready to compete in a game. She asks two kids to come up to the front of the room. Each kid is given a tube of toothpaste. Then, she says, whoever gets all of the toothpaste out the fastest will win a prize. And the kids are off, squeezing, using many techniques

---

[71] Marianne Spoon, "Training Compassion 'Muscle' May Boost Brain's Resilience to Others' Suffering," *W News* (blog), *University of Wisconsin-Madison*, May 22, 2018.

to get the last bit out as quickly as possible. The other kids are screaming, cheering, and shouting instructions. The whole thing takes on a life of its own.

But then, Teressa flips the script on the kids. "Okay," she says, "to win the game, now you have to get all the toothpaste back into the tube." She gives them each five minutes. The kids start trying, desperately to get the paste back in. They're using pencils, then their hands, then trying to manipulate the tube itself. But no matter what happens, no one can ever get the toothpaste back in.

"This toothpaste represents your words. It's why you need to be kind. Because words, once said, can never be taken back."

It may seem opportunistic to be kind to others to build your own resilience, but the truth is that kindness is truly contagious. According to a study from the University of Otago in New Zealand, small acts of kindness intended to benefit victims after a tragedy also appear to strengthen the resilience and wellbeing of the person performing the act of kindness. After the Christchurch terrorist attacks where more than forty-nine people were killed in a mosque, many people donated home-cooked meals, sent flowers, and performed other acts of condolence for family members of survivors and to honor the deceased. The New Zealand researchers found that these acts of kindness benefited both the giver and the receiver.[72]

In the paper's conclusion, the authors sum up their findings: "In times of challenge and tragedy, it can be easy to

---

72 Jill G. Hayhurst, John A. Hunter, and Ted Ruffman, "Encouraging Flourishing Following Tragedy: The Role of Civic Engagement in Well-Being and Resilience," *New Zealand Journal of Psychology* 48, no. 1 (April 2019) 75-94.

consider our own wellbeing as unimportant or trivial, especially compared to those who directly suffered from the terror attack. We argue, based on the literature and the results from the present study, that contributing to society and supporting our own wellbeing are two sides of the same coin—by being engaged and contributing, we bolster our wellbeing and become more resilient."

The truth is, there's never enough kindness in the world, and I probably don't have to convince you why it's important. But it's a tool we can use to help strengthen our own resilience, and empower those around us too.

CHAPTER 14

AUTHENTICITY

In my sophomore year of college, I decided I wanted to join a sorority. I almost did, until I started the rush process, which became one of the most awkward, yet defining, experiences of my life. I was moments away from trying to convince a group of strangers, my *peers*, that I was cool enough to hang out with them. Never did I think this moment would help to define my values for the entirety of my future.

Although I already had a good group of friends, I liked the idea of expanding my social network and having access to some of the best parties on campus. However, a few days before rush, I started to get cold feet. Something about the experience wasn't sitting well with me. I'd been given my instructions. I'd be placed in a cohort of other first- and second-year girls and we'd traipse through sorority houses and meet with the different organizations. Many of my friends were joining, and my need for community was strong. But I was dealing with internal conflict as I went over the process in my mind. In just a few minutes, these women, only one to three years older than me, were going to evaluate my fitness to join their social club.

They were sizing me up, seeing if I was made of the right material to hang out with them. For three days, I stewed about my decision to rush. In the end, I decided it wasn't for me. It felt like speed-dating for friends, with little more than looks to use as an evaluation tool. This felt too unnatural.

On the day of rush, I got a call from my pledge mom, the upperclassman who'd been assigned to my cohort of rushees. "Where are you? We're waiting for you and can't wait to meet you!" she exclaimed. I was embarrassed. I thought I could simply not show up to the event and I'd have automatically opted out of the process. But my rush mom was concerned for my wellbeing. I told her about my hesitation and that I didn't think I was sorority material. She was kind and offered up what I thought was a compelling solution. "I get it. But if you don't rush, then you don't have the option to pledge at all. You can always back out later if it's not for you."

I was somewhat convinced. I was laying in my bed, lazing around on a Saturday afternoon, but I could probably get myself together and get down there before they started.

"I'm in my pajamas, though, I'd need time to get ready," I said.

"Well, go into your closet and find your best outfit, and get your makeup on. Then, come on down! We'll be waiting for you!"

I hung up the phone. Something about that comment hit me in the gut. The fact that I needed to put on my best outfit for a bunch of girls so they could decide whether I was worthy of being their friend was the sign I needed. I decided the sorority life wasn't for me.

I called my rush mom back and told her I wouldn't be attending, and that was the end. I ended up with a solid group of friends in college, all of which I met organically.

Although the sorority life wasn't for me, I certainly saw the value and role it played in many of my friends' college lives.

I didn't realize then that I had a clear need for authenticity in my life. I've never been a fan of networking. In business school, I walked out of a seminar on how to expand your business network. The instructor was telling us how we needed to keep an excel sheet of all our contacts, friends, and colleagues alike, and keep tabs on how often we contacted them. "You should send them a note—a text or email—once quarterly, then check them off your list." He then shared how he interacted with a cousin of his via this technique, and how it eventually helped him get a job, "You never know what one connection will lead to."

I, feeling defiant, raised my hand.

"Isn't that incredibly disingenuous?" I quipped. The instructor told me it wasn't, and it was most important for us to keep tabs on our network. He said that networking was as much helping others as it was keeping tabs on them so they could help you. While I got the point, it made me feel uneasy. I wasn't sure I felt comfortable being told how to strategize the formation of genuine relationships with the intent of furthering my career.

So many people present themselves to the world in the way they think others would approve. They're searching for acceptance or looking for a way to fit in. Of course, it's appropriate to present ourselves in a socially acceptable manner, but by contorting our personalities into cookie cutter shapes, we can damage our individuality and, in turn, result in the masking of our true selves. According to Dr. Marcia Sirota, author, coach, and psychiatrist, not being true to ourselves can result in anxiety, depression, frustration, addiction, and a lack of meaning and fulfillment in our lives.[73]

Dr. Sirota shares that if you want to be more authentic, you have to first know yourself. That means getting in touch with your real feelings and having an understanding of your true values. Oftentimes, we tell stories of who we are and what we want to believe in. Many of us are simply playing out a fantasy from what we deemed as the "right thing to do." Those of us growing up without the encouragement of individuality were pressed to "fit in" from a very young age. The kids who were the most popular often lacked individuality or depth and were simply fitting the mold. So we grew up thinking we had to act a certain way and do certain things to achieve certain milestones.

Dr. Sirota also shares that when a person can discover who they really are and what they really want, they feel a sense of integration and wholeness within not only themselves but also in their relationships. When someone is genuine, people know and like the real person. But being authentic sometimes requires courage that might be hard to summon. We have to have the courage to be imperfect, and with that comes vulnerability.

When I reconnected with Trevor, much of our conversation circled around this concept of vulnerability and authenticity. Trevor had grown up as a mainstream boy in the eighties and early nineties, with a tough-guy persona. He, along with most boys his age, wasn't encouraged to share feelings. This continued throughout his high school experience, and even through college, particularly on the football field.

---

73 Marcia Sirota, "The Value of Authenticity: Being More Real and Identifying Those Who Aren't Real," *Authentic vs. Inauthentic* (blog), December 16, 2015.

Men weren't supposed to share how they felt. So he had to internalize any adverse feelings he had.

However, since Trevor's stroke and throughout his multitude of surgeries, he's found that his adversity and honesty about his illness can be an icebreaker for people, particularly for men. "I've found power in my voice. The more I share about my story, the more I can get out of someone else," he shared. By opening up about his past and his adversity, it allowed other people in his circle to, in turn, share their hardships. He's noticed that we all have them. By acknowledging our struggles, we destigmatize them for others.

Each Friday, Trevor and his work teammates have a happy hour to talk about non-work things and to connect in a more personal way. This even continued during the coronavirus lockdown in the spring of 2020. Each week, three people share a story about themselves, almost like a grown-up show-and-tell. At one point, it was Trevor's turn. He was anxious about sharing his story about his ulcerative colitis, stroke, and surgeries with his teammates. Would they be understanding? Would it be too much information?

During Trevor's show-and-tell, he shared with his coworkers his cane—the crutch he used for months after his stroke. He recounted how he relearned how to walk, struggled to talk, and endured months and months of physical therapy. He was met with overwhelming support and love. Out of the twenty people on the call, eighteen of them reached out in some way afterward to share how much his story had touched them, and how they were now in his corner. Everyone loved his message and felt his vulnerability.

Prior to Trevor's illness, he wasn't very comfortable sharing his personal life with others outside of his family. He credits the internalizing of his stressors as part of the reason his ulcerative colitis manifested. Stress about his job or marriage got the best of him and, ultimately, may have contributed to his illness. "I've found, post all this, that it's better to wear your emotions on your sleeve," he shares. "Everyone needs that outlet."

Trevor shared with me how important it is to be authentic, particularly as a dad. "I always encourage my son to share his feelings," he says. "When I was growing up, there were things I wasn't comfortable sharing with my parents. As a dad, I want him to share everything with me." Trevor also shared how important it is for his kids to go against the flow and feel comfortable with their authentic selves. But most importantly, to be sure they are the ones who have the confidence to pick others up, especially kids who are different. "It'd make me most proud to see them lift other kids up, to go against the flow."

Authenticity is about staying true to who you are and what you believe. It's not about your image. But achieving authenticity in a world with Instagram filters and contoured perfection makes that very hard and truly scary. Though the truth is, if you're more open about who you are, what you believe in, and what you stand for, you'll connect with people in a real way.

Bob Kegan, a professor at Harvard's School of Education, researches authenticity at work. In his book, *An Everyone Culture*, he shares that most people have two full-time jobs. The first is their regular job and the second, taking up an equal amount of time, is the additional job of managing their image and how they are perceived. In other words, they are trying to ensure positive impressions while avoiding negative ones. Kegan's research suggests that this "image protection" effort is causing serious psychological and physical stress.[74]

We can mitigate some of that stress, however, by increasing our authenticity. To be authentic, we must have the courage to be vulnerable. It's important to remember that vulnerability is the greatest measure of courage. We typically find courage and strength in other people's vulnerability, but when engaging with our own vulnerability, we tend to feel a combination of abject terror and insecurity.[75]

To be our most resilient selves, we must welcome vulnerability into our lives. Below, I've included some excellent tips from the Human Capital Institute to help grow into our authenticity by embracing vulnerability each day, both at work and in our personal lives.

- Be present. Avoid distractions, especially when in the presence of others.
- Listen. Truly listen; don't think about your response until it's your turn.
- Allow others' experiences and choices to be different than your own. Embrace them. Consider them.
- Accept more. Judge less.
- Do not parse people. Recognize people as their whole selves, not as parts of pieces.
- Recognize you are not alone—many people share your experience. Overcoming the shame of silence and keeping our experience in darkness requires vulnerability, and it builds community.

---

[74] Jennifer Eggers, "Authenticity, the Catalyst to Building Resilience," *Leader Shift Insights* (blog), November 16, 2019.

[75] "Vulnerability: The Courageous Cornerstone of Authenticity, Leadership," *Human Capital Institute* (blog), June 18, 2018.

- Step out of your comfort zone. Be brave enough to tell your story and role model vulnerability. In doing so, you make it safer for others.
- Remember that you are not your past; adversity is the very best catalyst for change and growth.

No shame exists in being honest and emotional. These are the gifts of what it means to be human.[76]

In every conversation I've had while writing this book, I've been blown away by the confidence these Thrivers have exuded when talking about their darkest moments. We've discussed everything from deep depression to bathroom accidents to relationship failures. These moments connected me even closer to each of these spectacular humans. While I was inspired by their resilience, their humility in defeat and darkness is what I've grown to admire most. Living with authenticity has liberated each of us in a very real way, and, in turn, has bolstered our confidence, strengthened our relationships, and improved our resilience exponentially.

---

[76] Marcia Sirota, ibid.

CHAPTER 15

BEING BETTER

In reflecting on my experiences while writing this book, I dove deep into my emotions and those of the people I interviewed. In doing so, I realized there were a few things that people who haven't experienced similar trauma don't quite understand. In an effort to share perspective, I want to reflect on two things. The first is how important it is to retain some semblance of normalcy, particularly as it involves friendships and relationships. In more direct terms, no matter my struggle, I still want to be there for the ones I love. It helps me feel more connected to them and, in turn, makes me feel whole.

When I was diagnosed, despite how closely I'd kept the information between my family and Janine, I knew I'd eventually need to share the news more broadly. For those closest to me, I'd find a time when we could be alone, and I'd share with them my diagnosis and prognosis. Their reactions varied. Some people knew exactly what to say and were kind and comforting. Others were at a loss for words, a completely normal reaction that I expect and certainly cannot fault. But in each of these conversations, I knew it would behoove me to be strong, to feel strong, and to look optimistic. This attitude would put the other person at ease and make the conversation easier for both of us.

Stephanie was living in North Carolina at the time of my diagnosis. At this point, we'd been friends for over twenty years, but we hadn't lived in the same town since high school. Regardless, we'd always made it a point to prioritize each other and would visit when we could. I was even the maid of honor at her wedding, which was one of the most beautiful days I can remember.

One week into my diagnosis, I got a text from Stephanie. She wanted to talk. It'd been a few weeks, or even months, since we'd chatted. I had been waiting for a time to talk to her but hadn't figured out quite what to say yet. Stephanie was a very busy person. At this point, she had two kids. She was working as a registered dietitian and was also working on an advanced certification in diabetes management. If we needed to chat, we'd have to make an appointment.

A week later, we finally caught each other. Talking to Stephanie is one of the easiest things I do in my life. We've been through so much together, growing up as young, silly kids sneaking out at night, navigating colleges, and dealing with struggle, loss, and love. Stephanie and I have always been able to talk about all of these things with ease. Even at this point, with the impending bomb I was about to drop, I felt calm.

And then, she said, "I have some news."

I waited for her, noticing a hint of excitement in her voice.

"I'm pregnant!"

My heart sunk. In one moment, I was at a complete loss of words. My lovely friend whose life was rolling along at the perfect pace, in the seemingly perfect marriage, with two perfect kids, a gorgeous house, and a great career, was pregnant again. I stalled, imagining the divergence in emotion we were each feeling in that moment. Her, thrilled with her beautiful, wonderful news, and me with my bombshell. Her with her glowing, glorious life, and mine about to be cut short. I was about to downpour on her parade.

After congratulations, I mustered up the courage to share my news. I told her I had been diagnosed with terminal cancer, my life expectancy was down to a couple of years, I couldn't ever have children, and my entire future had been cut short. She was quiet. And then, she simply said, "I love you."

I'll never forget that conversation and how I trumped Stephanie's incredible, glorious news with my sour, rotten, garbage cancer diagnosis. I'm not sure I navigated the conversation correctly, but I knew I had to tell Stephanie what was going on in my life, and she had to do the same. We somehow waffled back and forth between congratulations and joy to uncertainty and frustration. But I knew with most other people, it wouldn't always flow so easily.

As with a lot of patients, I received a ton of support when I became more comfortable talking about my illness with others. Once I mustered up the courage to start sharing, I was blown away by the support and love I started to receive. About three months into my treatment, I went public about my illness and opened up about my treatment plan and my fears on social media. The response was overwhelming. Once I shared my story, I was heartened by the droves of kindness and positive words I'd received. People offered to share their time, drive me to appointments, and bring me food. I experienced the ultimate silver lining.

A newer friend of mine ended up being an unlikely source of support and comfort during my treatment. Ashley and I had been friends for years, and she was a common confidant during my early months of chemo. We'd chat for hours about our relative fears in life, common goals, and exciting happenings. She was as comfortable talking about the fun things in life to keep me distracted as she was listening to my fears about the future. She was the most perfect companion and became a prominent part of my recovery team.

However, things changed when my treatment plan got a little bit harder. Two years after my initial diagnosis, my doctors and I decided to get more aggressive than we'd originally planned. We decided to go after my original tumor site just in case there was any residual cancer left after two years of treatment. We planned for both surgery and radiation, despite not finding cancer on any of my scans. Although it was a potentially pointless plan of attack, both my oncology team and I felt good about treating my cancer aggressively, as if I was an early stager. Luckily, our instincts were right. My surgeon cut me open and, sure enough, we found three millimeters of invasive cancer boldly hanging on. She snatched it out with clear margins.

Afterward, I completed a month of radiation to ensure any abnormal cells were wiped out. The entire process resurfaced a lot of my fears about cancer treatment, and I, accordingly, harbored a lot of stress and anxiety. The three months of planning, surgery, radiation, and recovery proved to be immensely stressful. I was lucky to have friends and family to count on that could, once again, step up to make me feel better when managing this never-ending illness.

Suddenly, however, Ashley was nowhere to be found. Over the past few months, I noticed she stopped calling and texting. She avoided me at parties and averted eye contact when we were near each other. Her distance from me was tangible, but I didn't know what to do. I was undergoing a stressful treatment regimen and didn't want to add anxiety to my life. Instead of confronting Ashley, I simply let her go. We stopped talking almost completely.

A few months later, Ashley invited me over for a glass of wine out of the blue. I was surprised but excited to spend some time with her. Although it felt like she had dropped me at a time when I was vulnerable, I still cared for her. I hoped we could rectify things in time. After a few glasses, our conversation started to shift from light and airy to more serious. That's when she finally got real.

I learned that evening that Ashley and her husband were trying to have children. I had known this, of course, but I didn't know they'd been trying for several years, and Ashley had several recent, scary complications. My heart broke for her, and I immediately consoled her. While I didn't know what it felt like to lose a pregnancy, I could empathize with her pain and frustration.

And then Ashley looked up at me through tear-filled eyes. "How am I supposed to talk about this with you? It's just a baby, not cancer, not my life that's at risk."

I realized then why Ashley had been avoiding me. She was dealing with very real emotions related to her complications. She felt like she couldn't confide in me because I'd compare my problems with hers. "It's not the same as having a terminal diagnosis," she said.

But that didn't mean Ashley's struggle wasn't real, and I couldn't be sympathetic to her pain. In fact, the minute she confided in me, her authenticity tugged at my heart. I knew how much she and her husband wanted children, and each month that went on without a pregnancy eroded their confidence. The agony, sadness, anger, and frustration must have been overwhelming, and I could empathize with each of these sentiments. Not because my pain was greater than hers or that I had gone through something *harder*, but because regardless of the level of pain, I knew what it felt to truly hurt.

Ashley admitted to me she'd been distant because she felt her struggles couldn't compare to mine. I'd also bet it would be hard to take on someone else's pain when you're dealing with your own, so I imagine Ashley's avoidance helped to protect the struggle she was managing in her own heart. I'm glad she was able to, eventually, share her fears with me. Pain cannot be compared, and I will never fault her for feeling any amount of bitterness, frustration, or downright anger. In fact, I could only share one thing with her: neither of our struggles were *our fault*. Sometimes, bad things just happen. Despite our differences in mourning, or the feelings of loss, or the depression we'd endured, the fact that we'd both been dealt a shitty hand was enough to find common ground. For us, that common denominator is the glue that sealed our friendship back together.

In contrast, since day one, Stephanie and I have found solace in one another's adversities. While Stephanie's pregnancy was a breeze, her complicated delivery left Benson with multiple medical conditions. Despite our differences in adversity, we found comfort in sharing challenges and stories. Our lives couldn't be more different, yet we are both fighting a seemingly unending battle. Our authenticity with each other and strong connection helped us to find solace in one another, simply in our wills to fight, versus the commonality of our struggle.

Both of these people are important, lasting figures in my life. We each have struggles that dictate our lives despite their differences. The exercise of comparing adversity is simply fruitless and doesn't help anyone. Despite the significance of our challenges, we all need support, we all need comfort, and we all need love.

My second big revelation while writing this book was how empathetic I'd become to those dealing with adversity. I'd learned where to be sensitive, what words to say to make someone feel better, and what things could potentially be interpreted as hurtful. Not everyone has the opportunity to gather so many insights on those who'd managed such hurt in their lives, and for the greater good, I started collecting some tips. I decided we all need to be a little more empathetic and have a better understanding of what it feels like to deal with adversity. So I wanted to share how each of us can be a better friend, companion, and support to those facing adversity.

A couple of months into my terminal diagnosis, I was still navigating how to talk about it with other people. It felt so awkward. I'd start point-blank, "I have stage four breast cancer."

"Oh! I heard that breast cancer is the most curable cancer you can get! Are you going to have a mastectomy?"

"No, it's stage four, so, incurable."

"But my friend had breast cancer and she just did chemo and radiation and then it went away."

"Yeah, but, mine's stage four. It's already metastasized into my lymph nodes, to my bloodstream, and into my liver."

"But I heard of someone that just…"

The rest of that sentence varies depending on how insistent they'd become. I'd receive stories of someone's brother's mother-in-law's best friend who had some kind of cancer but *beat it*. The beginning remained the same and the outcome was generally good. When talking with friends and family about my diagnosis, they'd always share their anecdotes, share what they'd read on the internet, or even share a story of someone they knew who had beaten the odds. I did appreciate their positivity, but the interaction always left me on the defensive. Why couldn't they simply acknowledge how difficult *my situation* was?

A few times, people in my life made my illness about them. Those were some of the hardest conversations I've ever had.

A few months into chemotherapy but before I had shared it publicly, one of my friends told a group of mutual acquaintances about my illness. Shortly thereafter, my mom was approached by someone at our local grocery store: one of the mothers of these acquaintances. Obviously, my mom was struggling with how to manage my illness, how to deal with her feelings, and the uncertainty of the diagnosis. We hadn't discussed our family's narrative, and there was still so much we didn't know. A woman asked about me and my treatment plan, and what we were going to do next. My mom was totally taken aback and left with a loss of words.

I, too, was still dealing with and learning how to understand my new normal. I hadn't yet figured out how to talk about it with people outside of my immediate support circle. After my mom's run-in, I also started to receive emails and Facebook messages out of the blue. I wasn't ready to respond or even constructively acknowledge my illness. And the notifications just stressed me out further.

Some people don't realize that it's actually very hard to accept communications about illness if you're not ready. This seems to be a common thread among Thrivers. We have this innate need to put the other person at ease and respond to them with hope and strength. This makes everyone more comfortable and creates a more positive exchange. At this point, I was still grappling with my faith. I didn't have a plan for my mental wellbeing. I didn't have my illness elevator pitch ready for public consumption.

I was furious. I could not believe my friend had shared my news, my personal, heartbreaking news before I had even come to terms with it. Now, I was managing messages from people everywhere without feeling equipped to handle the responses. I lashed out at her over text, incredulous that she'd taken it upon herself to use my illness to gain sympathy within her circle of friends. Throughout our conversation, I SCREAMED WITH ALL CAPS that this wasn't her news to share and I was still working on how to come to terms with my new normal. Her response stopped me dead in my tracks: "This is hard for me too, you know."

The anger I felt in that moment was indescribable. It felt as if my ears were releasing steam and my heart was thumping a million miles a minute. I was dealing with so many heartbreaking emotions, from the potential of my shortened life to my inability to have a family. In one instant, I had lost everything. My friend had just made my illness *about her*.

It didn't take her long to apologize. But it did take me a long time to understand why she did it.

The truth is, this friend took on my illness as her own. This was one of the most traumatic things that had happened in either of our lives. She felt my pain. She empathized with my uncertainty. She felt deeply about my shortened future. The problem is, she directed her grief in the wrong direction in that moment and that was at *me*.

Clinical Psychologist Susan Silk knows what it's like to be the recipient of inappropriate comments about her own illness. When she was hospitalized with a life-threatening illness, one of her colleagues complained about how hard the ordeal was for *her too*. The colleague wasn't wrong, illnesses almost always affect many more people than just the sick person.[77]

The problem is, shifting the spotlight away from the patient, or person in crisis, is unhelpful and hurtful. When sharing grief, the last thing you want to hear is someone else's story and how your grief is affecting them. Yet humans naturally tend to want to sympathize despite its lack of productivity. So the ill person becomes the comforter. This is not helpful.

After Susan recovered, she was inspired to create the Ring Theory, which is a model of caring that clearly outlines appropriate comfort based on proximity to the person in need. The basic idea is to "comfort in, dump out."

Here's how it works. Imagine concentric circles similar to a bull's eye. At the center of the bull's eye is the person or people directly affected by trauma, illness, or adversity. In the next closest ring is the person's caregiver—their spouse, children, or loving friend who is their closest confidant. In the next ring are more close friends, relatives, or neighbors. As you move outward toward more distant rings, closeness to the affected person is diminished.

The rule of the ring is simple: Comfort IN, Dump OUT.

If you're in the center ring, it sucks. You're managing pain and frustration and uncertainty, but you also have the right to complain to anybody. That means, every person outward from you is an acceptable earpiece about your trauma.

But once you move outward, there are rules of comfort. Your second ring, which includes your spouse or closest

---

[77] Elana Premack Sandler, "Ring Theory Helps Us Bring Comfort In," *Psychology Today* (blog), May 30, 2017.

family member or friend, is also managing frustration, anger, and uncertainty. They're allowed to feel scared and anxious about your illness. And they're allowed to voice those frustrations. But they have to do it outward. They can dump emotions out, but not in. They should never complain to the person in the center ring how tough their life is *because of them*. This doesn't mean their pain isn't real. It simply means they need to direct it appropriately.

I realize now how much my friend took on when she found out I was sick. We'd been friends for decades, and she witnessed how my illness could change a life in an instant. She was traumatized and she needed someone to lean on. That person, however, couldn't be me.

I've developed a thick skin over the years and have looked to humor and optimism to help manage my illness. Dallas agrees and uses the same tactic. That being said, the years of struggle and uncertainty have also helped us both be more sensitive to how people, and their respective communities, react to adversity. Despite my illness, I want my friends to share their struggles with me. I want to know what's affecting them daily. I know how to respond and react because of my experience with trauma and adversity. I also know what can be incredibly hurtful and that one well-meaning comment can send someone spiraling. Human connection and community are so important in healing, but we've got to do it right.

Dallas says, "I also openly tell people they can talk to me and complain to me because everything is relative. Oftentimes, people tell me they don't want to come off complaining about an injury or something because I have experienced something so much worse and am paralyzed and disabled.

I don't want this to be the case. When people are close to me, I want to know what they are going through or feeling."

In truth, we can all be better supporters. If you're reading this, maybe you're dealing with some adversity and some of these will resonate with you. But even more likely, you'll be the source of love and care for someone else who will be battling trauma or illness. There's no road map for how to be a good friend, but I have found that we Thrivers have a lot in common when it comes to our needs for support. Therefore, I've compiled a list of things to consider when talking to someone dealing with trauma or adversity.

1. **Try not to talk to them about someone you know who has the same affliction or illness unless their situation is *exactly the same or worse* and now, they are doing as well as them or better.** As a stage four breast cancer patient, I couldn't relate to stories about someone who was stage two and now thriving. If you know someone battling a disease, understand their subtype and grade before sharing success stories. I found myself feeling consistently defensive, reminding people my subtype was different, I was sicker, or I had worse odds. Sometimes they'd share a story about someone with a completely different kind of cancer, not understanding how different treatment protocols and survivability odds were across the diagnoses. I'd have to correct them, and it made me, and them, feel immeasurably worse.

2. This may sound like a no-brainer, but you'd be surprised at how often this one happens. **Don't talk about someone who has died from the illness they're managing.** Once going public about my diagnosis, a former

classmate of mine sent me a note about his aunt who had recently died from breast cancer. I understand that people want to connect with you when you're dealing with trauma and that human nature is to try and find commonalities. But keep the poor outcomes to yourself. I'm not sure if he wanted to somehow share in my mourning or grief, but it was one of the most unhelpful comments I'd received.

3. **Don't put expectations on their progress or outcome.** "People assume I'll just get better from here and recover," Dallas said. "I can do a million hours of physical therapy, but that doesn't mean a muscle or nerve that doesn't work is going to just suddenly start working. I can only work and strengthen to a certain degree what I can move. While everyone is well-intentioned, you almost feel like you are going to let people down if you don't have some miraculous recovery." In other words, stay positive, but let the Thriver guide their own expectations.

4. **As much as you want to, try not to overly bright-side them.** Just because someone is complaining, it doesn't always require a retort or solution. When I was first diagnosed, I often received comments of optimism, like "it could always be worse," or "at least you're doing well now." Immediately going to the bright side can sometimes feel like our pain needs to be fixed, and that wallowing is an unacceptable coping strategy. Sometimes, just saying, "I'm so sorry; I'm here if you need me" is more helpful than anything else.

5. Don't *just* say, **"What can I do to help?"** While this is completely well-intentioned, people who are facing illness or trauma often can't begin to organize requests

for help or are too embarrassed to do so. Instead, ask their spouse or primary caregiver what you could do to make their lives better. Or take it upon yourself to send them something useful like a meal or gift card to show you care.

6. Try not to ask or dwell on **why this happened**. I can't stress this enough. It's over; it happened. Dwelling on how or why I got cancer won't make it go away. In fact, it'll just make me feel worse, like I did something wrong, like I caused it. Don't ask me if it runs in my family (it doesn't), or if I was on birth control (none of your business), or if I drank dairy milk growing up (I didn't, not that it matters). Try not to search for a cause for the illness; it's irrelevant. Stephanie is used to this too. "I think people search for a reason why something happened so they can find comfort and assure themselves that the same won't happen to them," she said.

7. **It's okay to acknowledge the bad.** Dallas says, "There is a great quote that says, 'Just because someone carries it well doesn't mean it isn't heavy.' There are so many things that I deal with daily that really suck. Even though I am doing extremely well and like to hide most things from people not everything is all rosy." While keeping things light and positive can be a good coping strategy, allowing someone to be real with you about what truly sucks can go a really long way.

8. **Don't ignore them.** Probably the worst thing you can say to someone managing trauma is nothing at all. A handful of people in my life have simply ignored my illness. I know it's not because they don't care about me, but probably because they're at a loss for words. In fact, I am sure some of them are following me and my

journey and are cheering me on, albeit silently. But if someone you know, even distantly, is managing crisis and has shared their struggles publicly, tell them you're thinking about them, send them a card, or reach out to them in some way. Even if you think it's been too long or you're not quite sure what to say, saying nothing is most certainly the most hurtful thing you can do.

If you're reading this list and feeling defensive, don't worry. These are common things we all do to try and connect with the people in our lives who are struggling. You're well-intended, and we know your love is honest and true. But the thing is, all you need to do is say you love them, or you care about them, or you're there for them. Even better, actually be *there* for them. Thrivers are so uniquely resilient that they don't need big, grand gestures; they just want to know you care. And I bet they're the most empathetic, open-minded listeners you'll find when you have something to vent about, no matter the size of your struggle.

***

Building resilience is an important part of growth and change for all of us. Over the years, I've faced a level of adversity that has, in part, taught me how to look forward with optimism, not behind in fear or regret. I believe this vantage point has not only helped me to thrive but has also given me better odds to survive. All the Thrivers in this book have built stronger lives since their trauma, but not because they're ignoring their challenges; they're emboldened by them. Life is sweeter when you truly know what's at risk.

You may not have faced the trauma level of the Thrivers in this book, but I'm certain you've faced adversity in your life. I challenge you now to use that to your advantage. Use nutrition and exercise as tools for your body and mind. Shape your mindset to find the good in the world. Love openly and honestly. Spread kindness like wildfire. Live your most authentic life. Use these tools to build upon your resilience every day.

I'm positive that you can withstand any storm.

"The oak fought the wind and was broken, the willow bent when it must and survived."
—ROBERT JORDAN, *THE FIRES OF HEAVEN*[78]

---

78 Robert Jordan, *The Fires of Heaven* (New York: Tor Books, 1994), 617.

ACKNOWLEDGMENTS

I never thought I'd write a book so deeply personal, but when I began to talk about my journey battling cancer, I couldn't help but include the details and stories of my life that made me who I am. Cancer isn't my defining characteristic, but it has helped me explore parts of my life I'd ignored or repressed over the years. This process has been nothing short of cathartic.

This story, however, is most certainly enhanced by the dialogues I had and the stories I received from Thrivers. Trevor, Nancy, Dallas, Kate, Stephanie, and Teressa—you all have given me the gift of your time, your story, and your authenticity. This book, and my life, will forever be enhanced by our conversations.

To Janine, Mom, and Dad: Your love and support have been the backbone of my resilience. Without you, I'd never be able to thrive with a terminal illness.

To Emily, Carmen, Beth, and Shelby: Thank you for letting me bounce ideas and stories off you, for your candor and understanding, and your unwavering support.

To Michael, Bill, Evan, Barbara, Lauren, Jojo, Fabienne, Janine M., Leslie, Rachel E., Carly, Xavier, Christina, Chancey, Leah, Jen, Adam, and Rachel R.: Thank you for your commitment to my success, and your detailed thoughts and insights about my book. You've each enhanced it immeasurably.

To Erik Koester, Chelsea Friday, Jordan Waterwash, and New Degree Press: Thank you for all your insights and motivation, and for helping me bring my dream into reality.

Finally, thank you to everyone who helped spread the word about *Nourishing Resilience* to gather momentum and help me publish a book I am proud of. I am sincerely grateful for all your help.

APPENDIX

Introduction

American Cancer Society. "Cancer Facts and Figures 2020." Accessed September 1, 2020. https://www.cancer.org/research/cancer-facts-statistics/all-cancer-facts-figures/cancer-facts-figures-2020.html.

Center for Disease Control. "Learn about Mental Health." Accessed August 28, 2020. https://www.cdc.gov/mentalhealth/learn/index.htm.

Tedeschi, Richard and Lawrence Calhoun. "Posttraumatic Growth: Conceptual Foundations and Empirical Evidence." *Psychological Inquiry* 15, 1 (2004): 1-18. https://www.semanticscholar.org/paper/Posttraumatic-Growth%3A-Conceptual-Foundations-and-Tedeschi-Calhoun/9948d303099caa7915eb23da1df89602f70a0f1d.

Chapter 1

American Psychological Association. "Building Your Resilience." Accessed May 15, 2020. https://www.apa.org/topics/resilience.

Joshi, Deepak, Tobias Dickel, Rakesh Aga, and Gray Smith-Laing. "Stroke in Inflammatory Bowel Disease: A Report of Two Cases and Review of the Literature." *Thrombosis Journal* 6, 2 (2008). https://thrombosisjournal.biomedcentral.com/articles/10.1186/1477-9560-6-2.

Southwick, Stephen M., George A. Bonanno, Ann S. Masten, Catherine Panter-Brick, and Rachel Yehuda. "Resilience Definitions, Theory, and Challenges: Interdisciplinary Perspectives." *European Journal of Psychotraumatology* 5, 1 (October 2014): 25338. https://www.ncbi.nlm.nih.gov/pmc/articles/PMC4185134/.

Vitelli, Romeo. "Learning to be Resilient." *Psychology Today,* May 13, 2013. https://www.psychologytoday.com/us/blog/media-spotlight/201305/learning-be-resilient.

Chapter 2

American Cancer Society. "Cancer Facts and Figures 2020." Accessed August 20, 2020. https://www.cancer.org/research/cancer-facts-statistics/all-cancer-facts-figures/cancer-facts-figures-2020.html.

BrainLine (blog). "What Is the Glasgow Coma Scale?" February 13, 2018. Accessed August 30, 2020. https://www.brainline.org/

article/what-glasgow-coma-scale#:~:text=The%20Glasgow%20Coma%20Scale%20(GCS,of%20an%20acute%20brain%20injury.

BreastCancer.org. "Risk of Developing Breast Cancer." Accessed September 6, 2020. https://www.breastcancer.org/symptoms/understand_bc/risk/understanding.

Keeton, Courtney Pierce, Maureen Perry-Jenkins, and Aline G. Sayer. "Sense of Control Predicts Depressive and Anxious Symptoms Across the Transition to Parenthood." *Journal of Family Psychology* 22, 2 (2008): 212-221. https://www.ncbi.nlm.nih.gov/pmc/articles/PMC2834184/.

Komen Perspectives (blog). "Does Pregnancy Affect Breast Cancer Risk and Survival?" January 2012. Accessed September 6, 2020. https://blog.komen.org/blog/komen-perspectives-does-pregnancy-affect-breast-cancer-risk-and-survival/.

Langer, E. J. and J. Rodin. "The Effects of Choice and Enhanced Personal Responsibility for the Aged: A Field Experiment in an Institutional Setting." *Journal of Personality and Social Psychology* 43, 2 (1976). https://pubmed.ncbi.nlm.nih.gov/1011073/.

Pagnini, Francisco, Katherine Bercovitz, and Ellen Langer. "Perceived Control and Mindfulness: Implications for Clinical Practice. *Journal of Psychotherapy Integration* 26, 2 (2016): 91-102. https://www.apa.org/pubs/journals/features/int-int0000035.pdf.

Chapter 3

Pagnini, Francisco, Katherine Bercovitz, and Ellen Langer. "Perceived Control and Mindfulness: Implications for Clinical Practice." *Journal of Psychotherapy Integration* 26, 2 (2016): 91-102. https://www.apa.org/pubs/journals/features/int-int0000035.pdf.

Slavich, George M. and Michael R. Irwin. "From Stress to Inflammation and Major Depressive Disorder: A Social Signal Transduction Theory of Depression." *Psychological Bulletin* 140, 3 (January 2014): 774-815. https://www.ncbi.nlm.nih.gov/pmc/articles/PMC4006295/.

Verma, Prakar. "How to Develop a Non-judgmental Attitude to Live More Peacefully." *The Startup* (blog), September 27, 2018. https://medium.com/swlh/how-to-stop-judging-and-start-living-91bef2834c9a.

Chapter 4

Collier, Lorna. "Growth after Trauma." *Monitor on Psychology* 47, 10 (November 2016): 48. https://www.apa.org/monitor/2016/11/growth-trauma.

Graves, Ginny. "Is There an Upside to Tragedy?" *Oprah* (blog), July 2015. http://www.oprah.com/inspiration/post-traumatic-growth/all.

Joseph, Stephen. "What Doesn't Kill Us." *The Psychologist* 25 (2012): 816-819. https://thepsychologist.bps.org.uk/volume-25/edition-11/what-doesnt-kill-us.

Relias Media. "Life Expectancy after Aortic Valve Replacement." Accessed June 12, 2020. https://www.reliasmedia.com/articles/144956-life-expectancy-after-aortic-valve-replacement#:~:text=During%20a%20median%206.8%20years,of%20age%20(4.4%20years).

Tedeschi, Richard and Lawrence Calhoun. "Posttraumatic Growth: Conceptual Foundations and Empirical Evidence." *Psychological Inquiry* 15, no. 1 (2004): 1-18. https://www.jstor.org/stable/20447194.

Chapter 5

Nelson, D. V., L. C. Friedman, P. E. Baer, M. Lane, and F. E. Smith. "Attitudes of Cancer: Psychometric Properties of Fighting Spirit and Denial." *Journal of Behavioral Medicine* 12, 4 (August 1989): 341-355. https://europepmc.org/article/med/2600963.

Nurmohame, Samir. "The Underdog Effect: When Low Expectations Increase Performance." *Academy of Management Journal* 63, 4 (August 24, 2020). https://journals.aom.org/doi/10.5465/amj.2017.0181.

Petticrew, Mark, Ruth Bell, and Duncan Hunter. "Influence of Psychological Coping on Survival and Recurrence in People with Cancer: Systematic Review." *BMJ* 325 (November 9, 2002). https://www.ncbi.nlm.nih.gov/pmc/articles/PMC131179/.

Chapter 6

American Heart Association News (blog). "What's Your Sense of Purpose? The Answer May Affect Your Health." October 8, 2019. Accessed September 1, 2020. https://www.heart.org/en/news/2019/10/08/whats-your-sense-of-purpose-the-answer-may-affect-your-health.

Boyle, Patricia A. "Effect of a Purpose in Life on Risk of Incident Alzheimer Disease and Mild Cognitive Impairment in Community-Dwelling Older Persons." *Archives of General Psychology* 67, 3 (March 2010): 304-310. https://www.ncbi.nlm.nih.gov/pmc/articles/PMC2897172/.

Buttner, Dan. "The Minnesota Miracle." *AARP Online* (blog). Accessed September 1, 2020. https://www.aarp.org/health/longevity/info-01-2010/minnesota_miracle.html.

Krause, Neal. "Meaning in Life and Mortality." *Journal of Gerontology Series B: Psychological Sciences and Social Sciences* 64, 4 (June 2009): 517-527. https://www.ncbi.nlm.nih.gov/pmc/articles/PMC2905132/.

Leonard, Barb and Mary Jo Kreitzer. "Why Is Life Purpose Important?" *Taking Charge of Your Health & Wellbeing* (blog). Accessed September 1, 2020. https://www.takingcharge.csh.umn.edu/why-life-purpose-important.

Mogi, Ken. "This Japanese Secret to a Longer and Happier Life is Gaining Attention from Millions Around the World." *Make It* (blog). *CNBC*, May 22, 2019. https://www.cnbc.com/2019/05/22/

the-japanese-secret-to-a-longer-and-happier-life-is-gaining-attention-from-millions.html.

Chapter 7

O'Riordan, Michael. "Younger Type 2 Diabetes Patients Face Higher Mortality and CVD Risks." *The Heart Beat* (blog). *TCTMD*, April 10, 2019. https://www.tctmd.com/news/younger-type-2-diabetes-patients-face-higher-mortality-and-cvd-risks.

Science Daily (blog). "Culture Influences Young People's Self Esteem: Fulfillment of Value Priorities of Other Individuals Important to Youth." February 14, 2014. Accessed September 2, 2020. https://www.sciencedaily.com/releases/2014/02/140224081027.htm.

Chapter 8

Brown, S. L., Randolph M. Nesse, Amiram D. Vinokur, and Dylan M. Smith. "Providing Social Support May Be More Beneficial Than Receiving It: Results from a Prospective Study of Mortality." *Psychological Science* 14, 4 (2003): 320-327. https://pubmed.ncbi.nlm.nih.gov/12807404/.

Plante, Thomas G. "Helping Others Offers Surprising Benefits." *Psychology Today* (blog). July 2, 2012. Accessed September 4, 2020. https://www.psychologytoday.com/us/blog/do-the-right-thing/201207/helping-others-offers-surprising-benefits-0.

Thoits, Peggy A. and Lyndi Hewitt. "Volunteer Work and Wellbeing." *Journal of Health and Societal Behavior* 42, 2 (June 2001):

115-131. https://www.asanet.org/sites/default/files/savvy/images/members/docs/pdf/featured/volunteer.pdf.

Van Der Linden, Sander. "The Helper's High." *Odewire* (blog). December 2011. Accessed September 2, 2020. https://scholar.princeton.edu/sites/default/files/slinden/files/helpershigh.pdf.

Chapter 9

Alipio, M. "Vitamin D Supplementation Could Possibly Improve Clinical Outcomes of Patients Infected with Coronavirus-2019 (COVID-2019)." *SSRN Electronic Journal* (2020). https://www.ncbi.nlm.nih.gov/pmc/articles/PMC7266578/.

Calder, Philip C. "Omega-3 Polyunsaturated Fatty Acids and Inflammatory Processes: Nutrition or Pharmacology?" *British Journal of Clinical Pharmacology* 75, no. 3 (February 2015): 645-662. https://pubmed.ncbi.nlm.nih.gov/22765297/.

Dian, Corneliussen-James. "Speaking Out on Metastatic Breast Cancer." *Metavivor* (blog). November 7, 2014. Accessed August 22, 2020. https://www.metavivor.org/blog/speaking-out-on-metastatic-breast-cancer/.

Hossein-nezhad, Arash, Avrum Spira, and Michael F. Holick. "Influence of Vitamin D Status and Vitamin D3 Supplementation on Genome Wide Expression of White Blood Cells: A Randomized Double-Blind Clinical Trial." *PloS One* 8, 3 (March 20, 2013). https://pubmed.ncbi.nlm.nih.gov/23527013/.

Kotepui, Manas. "Diet and Risk of Breast Cancer." *Contemporary Oncology* 20, 1 (2016): 13-19. https://www.ncbi.nlm.nih.gov/pmc/articles/PMC4829739/.

Michigan Medicine, University of Michigan. "Gastrointestinal Complications (PDQ): Supportive Care – Health Professional Information (NCI)." Accessed September 12, 2020. https://www.uofmhealth.org/health-library/ncicdr0000062834.

Mohebi-Nejad, Azin and Behnood Bikdeli. "Omega-3 Supplements and Cardiovascular Diseases." *Tanaffos Journal of Respiratory Diseases, Thoracic Surgery, Intensive Care, and Tuberculosis* 13, 1 (2014) 6-14. https://www.ncbi.nlm.nih.gov/pmc/articles/PMC4153275/.

The Nutrition Source (blog). "Vegetables and Fruits." *The Harvard T. H. Chan School of Public Health.* Accessed September 12, 2020. https://www.hsph.harvard.edu/nutritionsource/what-should-you-eat/vegetables-and-fruits/.

Paul, Bidisha, Yuanyuan Li, and Trygve O. Tollefsbol. "The Effects of Combinatorial Genistein and Sulforaphane in Breast Tumor Inhibition: Role in Epigenetic Regulation." *International Journal of Molecular Sciences* 19, 6 (2018). https://pubmed.ncbi.nlm.nih.gov/29899271/.

Phaniendra, Alugoju, Dinesh Babu Jestadi, and Latha Periyasamy. "Free Radicals: Properties, Sources, Targets, and Their Implication in Various Diseases." *Indian Journal of Clinical Biochemistry* 30, 1 (January 2015): 11-26. https://www.ncbi.nlm.nih.gov/pmc/articles/PMC4310837/.

Popkin, Barry M., Kristen E. D'Anci, and Irwin H. Rosenberg. "Water, Hydration and Health." *Nutrition Review* 68, 8 (August 2010): 439-458. https://www.ncbi.nlm.nih.gov/pmc/articles/PMC2908954/.

Chapter 10

Best, T. M. and C. A. Asplund. *DeLee, Drez, & Miller's Orthopaedic Sports Medicine,* 5th ed. Philadelphia, PA: Elsevier, 2020.

Betof, Alison S., Christopher D. Lascola, Douglas Weitzel, Chelsea Landon, Peter M. Scarbrough, Gayathri R. Devi, Gregory Palmer, Lee W. Jones, and Mark W. Dewhirst. "Modulation of Murine Breast Tumor Vascularity, Hypoxia, and Chemotherapeutic Response by Exercise." *Journal of the National Cancer Institute* 107, 5 (May 2015). https://pubmed.ncbi.nlm.nih.gov/25780062/.

Chapter 11

Cleveland Clinic. "Stress." Accessed September 8, 2020. https://my.clevelandclinic.org/health/articles/11874-stress.

Doll, Karen. "23 Resilience Boosting Tools and Exercises." *Positive Psychology* (blog). January 9, 2020. https://positivepsychology.com/resilience-activities-exercises/.

National Institutes of Mental Health. "5 Things You Should Know About Stress." Accessed September 8, 2020. https://www.nimh.nih.gov/health/publications/stress/19-mh-8109-5-things-stress_142898.pdf.

WebMD. "Stress Symptoms." Accessed September 8, 2020. https://www.webmd.com/balance/stress-management/stress-symptoms-effects_of-stress-on-the-body.

Chapter 12

CBS News (blog). "Holding Spouse's Hand May Reduce Stress." December 20, 2006. Accessed August 22, 2020. https://www.cbsnews.com/news/holding-spouses-hand-may-reduce-stress/.

Charnetski, Carl J., and Francis X. Brennan. "Sexual Frequency and Salivary Immunoglobulin A (IgA)." *Psychological Reports* 94, 3 (1994): 839-844. https://pubmed.ncbi.nlm.nih.gov/15217036/.

Charnetski, Carl J., Sandra Riggers, and Francis X. Brennan. "Effect of Petting a Dog on Immune System Function." *Psychological Reports* 95, 3 (2004): 1087-1091. https://pubmed.ncbi.nlm.nih.gov/15762389/.

Holt-Lunstad, Julianne, Timothy B. Smith, and J. Bradley Layton. "Social Relationships and Mortality Risk: A Meta-Analytic Review." *PloS Medicine,* July 27, 2010. https://journals.plos.org/plosmedicine/article?id=10.1371/journal.pmed.1000316.

Mills, Harry and Mark Dombeck. "Resilience: Relationships." *Helen Farabee Centers* (blog). Accessed September 9, 2020. https://www.helenfarabee.org/poc/center_index.php?cn=298.

Natale, Nicol. "Falling in Love Changes Your Body and Brain – Here's How." *Business Insider* (blog). July 12, 2018. Accessed

August 25, 2020. https://www.sciencealert.com/falling-in-love-changes-your-body-and-brain-here-s-how.

National Institute on Aging. "Depression and Older Adults." Accessed September 8, 2020. https://www.nia.nih.gov/health/depression-and-older-adults.

Parker-Pope, Tara. "Love and Pain Relief." *Wellblogs* (blog), *The New York Times*. October 13, 2010. Accessed August 25, 2020. https://well.blogs.nytimes.com/2010/10/13/love-and-pain-relief/.

Chapter 13

Hayhurst, Jill G., John A. Hunter, and Ted Ruffman. "Encouraging Flourishing Following Tragedy: The Role of Civic Engagement in Wellbeing and Resilience." *New Zealand Journal of Psychology* 48, 1 (April 2019): 75-94. https://www.researchgate.net/publication/332769082_Encouraging_flourishing_following_tragedy_The_role_of_civic_engagement_in_wellbeing_and_resilience.

Spoon, Marianne. "Training Compassion 'Muscle' May Boost Brain's Resilience to Others' Suffering." *W News* (blog), *University of Wisconsin-Madison*, May 22, 2018. Accessed September 20, 2020. https://news.wisc.edu/training-compassion-muscle-may-boost-brains-resilience-to-others-suffering/.

Chapter 14

Eggers, Jennifer. "Authenticity, the Catalyst to Building Resilience." *Leader Shift Insights* (blog). November 16, 2019. Accessed September 20, 2020. https://leadershiftinsights.com/authenticity/.

Human Capital Institute (blog). "Vulnerability: The Courageous Cornerstone of Authenticity, Leadership." June 18, 2018. Accessed September 2, 2020. https://www.hci.org/blog/vulnerability-courageous-cornerstone-authenticity-leadership#:~:text=Vulnerability%3A%20The%20Courageous%20Cornerstone%20of%20Authenticity%2C%20Leadership,-Develop%20Your%20Workforce&text=The%20cultivation%20of%20vulnerability%20in,and%20develop%20comfort%20with%20ofailure.

Sirota, Marcia. "The Value of Authenticity: Being More Real and Identifying Those Who Aren't Real." *Authentic vs. Inauthentic* (blog). December 16, 2015. Accessed September 20, 2020. https://medium.com/@marciasirota/the-value-of-authenticity-being-real-and-identifying-those-who-aren-t-real-28f8ace03532.

Chapter 15

Jordan, Robert. *The Fires of Heaven*. New York: Tor Books, 1994.

Sandler, Elana Premack. "Ring Theory Helps Us Bring Comfort In." *Psychology Today* (blog), May 30, 2017. https://www.psychologytoday.com/us/blog/promoting-hope-preventing-suicide/201705/ring-theory-helps-us-bring-comfort-in.

Printed in Great Britain
by Amazon